WHEN SPIRITS COME CALLING

"It's wonderful! Well-written and on a topic that is full of fascination and hope for many people. I like the stance of skepticism, rather than thoughtless belief or closed-minded rejection. The reporting is clear and factual, and the stories themselves are enthralling."

—Mary Manin Morrissey, senior minister,
Living Enrichment Center, and
author, *Building Your Field of Dreams*

"Superbly written and well researched, *When Spirits Come Calling* [will] stimulate your thoughts about the afterlife. . . . It will open your heart to the wonder and mystery [of] spontaneous experiences involving deceased loved ones and the living."

—Louis E. LaGrand, Ph.D., Distinguished Service Professor
Emeritus, State University of New York,
and author, *Gifts from the Unknown*

"*When Spirits Come Calling* is a book I strongly recommend to all who still have an open mind about what happens to us after our demise. It is intelligent, open-minded and very readable."

—John Beloff, Ph.D., author, *Parapsychology:
A Concise History*; editor, *Journal of
the Society for Psychical Research*, 1982–1999

"Prof. Wright has conducted a serious investigation into an important human experience—after death contacts. In this ground-breaking book, you sense the author's sincere compassion for her interview subjects—a welcome contrast to more conventional studies that assume that people who experience such phenomena must be reacting irrationally to trauma, i.e., death of a loved one. Wright does not distort her subjects' accounts to make them fit the secular (atheistic) assumptions associated with so much contemporary science. A real gem, empirically bold, well-reasoned, yet humble in the face of a great mystery."

—Michael Dreiling, sociology professor,
University of Oregon

"The question of the survival of bodily death has been scientifically explored for more than a century. In *When Spirits Come Calling,* Prof. Wright skillfully documents her conclusion that something does indeed survive. Her probing interviews make it clear that seeing an apparition, or sensing the presence of a deceased loved one is not merely some kind of extrasensory perception, but rather is a genuine encounter with a surviving intelligence. I highly recommend this fascinating and carefully researched book."

—Russell Targ, physicist and parapsychologist,
co-author, *Miracles of Mind: Exploring
Nonlocal Consciousness and Spiritual Healing*

"Sylvia Hart Wright offers compelling evidence to us postmodern agnostics, atheists, and skeptics that we are not alone—and that is good news!"

—Charles Sturms, professor of intercultural
studies, Northwest Christian College,
and Disciples of Christ minister

"The world of science looks for proof by experimental findings and discounts anecdotal reports because of the very uniqueness of each report. However, the method of science begins with observation. Sylvia Hart Wright has taken an important first step. She has noticed the frequency with which people told of encounters with loved ones who had died. . . . [Their accounts] tell us something important and perhaps universal about human consciousness."

—Paula Bram Amar, Ph.D., consulting psychologist,
expert on biofeedback

"Contains a wealth of moving personal stories presented in an incomparably warmhearted yet cool-headed manner, and illuminated by the author's sensitive and searching cross-cultural analysis."

—Madronna Holden, Ph.D., anthropologist
and educator, Linfield College

When Spirits Come Calling

The Open-Minded Skeptic's Guide to After-Death Contacts

SYLVIA HART WRIGHT

with a foreword by
ANDREW M. GREELEY

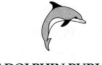

BLUE DOLPHIN PUBLISHING

Published by Blue Dolphin Publishing, Inc.
P.O. Box 8, Nevada City, CA 95959
Orders: 1-800-643-0765
Web: www.bluedolphinpublishing.com

ISBN: 1-57733-095-1 softcover
ISBN: 1-57733-125-7 hardcover

Library of Congress Cataloging-in-Publication Data

Wright, Sylvia Hart.
    When spirits come calling : the open-minded skeptic's guide to
after-death contacts / Sylvia Hart Wright ; with a foreword by
Andrew M. Greeley.
        p. cm.
    Includes index.
    ISBN 1-57733-095-1
    1. Spiritualism. 2. Bereavement—Psychological aspects. 3. Future
life. 4. Immortality. 5. Science and spiritualism. I. Title.

BF1261.2 .W75 2001
133.9—dc21
                                                        2001035831

First edition, April 2002

Quotations from interviews are central to this book. These have been
edited for clarity and conciseness. Some names and other details have
been changed to protect anonymity. The author believes that, in every
other respect, the stories reported here are as authentic as sincere
informants can make them.

Printed in the United States of America

10   9   8   7   6   5   4   3   2   1

To Charles
and to all the sensitive and candid people
who believed that spirits had reached out to them
and who shared their stories with me.

Table of Contents

Foreword   xi

1. After-Death Contact—A Common Experience   1

2. Sensing Someone Else's Death   16

3. Knowledge and Guidance from the Other Side   31

4. How World Religions View Survival of the Spirit   47

5. Facing up to a Cultural Taboo   61

6. After a Suicide   77

7. Subtle Contacts—Scents and a Feeling of Closeness   92

8. After the Death of a Child   105

9. Lights That Blink a Message   115

10. Misbehaving Radios, Telephones—and More   124

11. Symbolic Events   136

12. Animal Stories   149

13. More Help and Guidance from Loving Spirits   159

14. Ghosts, Possession, and Things That Go Bump
    in the Night   172

15. What's So Different About Paranormal Dreams?   188

16. Who Becomes a Sensitive?   194

17. Spiritual Experience and Religious Belief   211

Notes   224

Index   235

About the Author   241

Foreword

A CERTAIN KIND OF "SCIENTIST" will reject all the stories reported by
Prof. Wright in this book. The dead do not return and that's that.
Therefore none of the stories are true. Since they cannot be true,
they must be the result of wish-fulfillment or fraud. Contact with
the dead is a pipe dream and ought not to be taken seriously in a
scientific age.

Yet some two out of five Americans report contact experiences. Certainly, as William James once wrote, those who have not
encountered the dead, have no obligation to accept the judgment
of those who say that such contacts are possible. On the other
hand, those who have "been there" do not have to accept the
"scientific" verdict on their experiences. The critics are forced by
their philosophy, not their science, to reject Wright's stories. They
are talking past those who have experienced them. They are rather
talking to themselves, often nervously.

Do I believe in contact with dead? In fact I do not. I believe in
God's implacably forgiving love; I believe that God's love is stronger than death, that God would, as the poet Paul Murray puts it, die
of sadness if one of us should cease to exist. Contact with the dead
is not required for faith. Moreover faith should not depend on such
contact.

At best such experiences are, as Carol Zalesky describes them,
signs, hints of mystery, wonder and surprise in the cosmos, whose
mystery increases the more we seem to have rolled back mystery.

I accept as facts to be explained some incidents in which two separate persons have had the same experience, though they are not present to one another. Such stories, however, do no more than to persuade me that perhaps some of these experiences are possible. Because we wish something to be true, the fact of our wish does not make them false. I take it that such events do seem to occur and feel no need to account for them either metaphysically or theologically.

I wish that scientists would approach phenomena of the sort Prof. Wright describes with more open minds. I am embarrassed when a scientist closes his mind because he thinks something is impossible. It strikes me that it is immodest for a scientist to say that something did not happen because it could not have happened. It would be much better if he said something like, I don't think so, but I don't know for sure.

I wish my own sociological profession would admit that something which happens to 40% of Americans is at least interesting and explore the antecedents and the consequences of these events. In a recent survey of American medical doctors, a large majority felt that contact with the dead experiences in the death room were "clinically valid." I'm not sure what this means, but it does mean that the doctors have surely not set their minds against the possibility of death-room events.

Wright's critics will bitterly oppose her stories because they take it as obvious that there is no life after death. Her ardent supporters hope that there might be life after death, and hence they will support the stories as evidence that there are grounds for hope. Neither side will ever win the argument this side of paradise.

Those of us who know with the hesitant certainty of faith that God will not let his beloved children vanish into non-being will welcome the stories as signs, nothing more than hints perhaps, but nothing less either.

Andrew Greeley
Grand Beach
June 2001

WHEN SPIRITS COME CALLING

1

After-Death Contact—
A Common Experience

HAS SOMEONE YOU KNOW lost a beloved partner? If they confide that they've sometimes sensed their lost mate's presence, don't assume that grief has tipped them over the edge.

Studies by doctors, psychologists, social workers, and public opinion researchers confirm that experiences of apparent contact with the dead are commonplace all over the world. For instance, over half the healthy, normal widows and almost as large a percentage of widowers in the United States sense the presence of their departed mates at least once afterwards. Such experiences are usually unexpected and spontaneous, not invited in any way. They are also direct—they do *not* involve mediums.

Apparent contacts are most common in the first year after bereavement, but they may recur for years, even for decades. Most such visits from "beyond the veil" are perceived as pleasant. A significant few bring guidance or information that it would seem could only come from a spirit source.

This book documents over a hundred such contact experiences, as reported since 1998 by the normal, everyday folks who experienced them. The majority of them are not bereaved spouses. It's common for sane, active women and men to sense contact with their deceased parents or children, with grandparents, siblings or friends. But because more research has been done on widows and widowers—in England and Wales, Japan, Norway and Sweden, as

1

well as in the United States—it's easier to cite statistics about their experiences. In 1983 I myself was widowed. Soon I was confronted by mysteries unlike any I'd ever imagined.

HOW THE ADVENTURE BEGAN FOR ME

I was well into my forties—a college professor and the published author of a scholarly book about contemporary architecture—when a startling event forced me to ponder whether spirits can survive and contact the living. Since then, further personal experiences plus lots of research have taught me that the death of the body is not the end of all consciousness. Instead, it's a doorway to something else.

When I was widowed in 1983, I had been married for ten years to Paul Fletcher. It was not a first marriage for either of us. Paul was a warm and loving man, supportive to me and cheerfully committed to helping me raise my young son, Keith, from a previous marriage. Paul was also an outspoken atheist but that hardly bothered me since I had considered myself an agnostic for as long as I'd understood the meaning of the word.

When we married in New York, Paul was a tall and vigorous 51 year-old with a wild and sometimes salty sense of humor, and a linguist's delight in wordplay. As Keith and I picked up his verbal addiction, the three of us often sat laughing around our dinner table, circling it with a sequence of ever more outrageous puns. With Paul's barrel chest and lots of wavy brown hair lightly flecked with gray, my bluff, gregarious husband looked a decade younger. But diabetes, which he'd had for some twenty years, was gnawing away at him from within. Two years after our wedding at the Unitarian-Universalist church where we had met—a humanistic church that had no creed which we could not sincerely affirm—a massive hemorrhage caused by diabetic retinopathy destroyed the vision of his right eye. For two more years he got by reasonably well until, in November of 1977, a smaller hemorrhage damaged his other eye.

Now he was legally blind. By profession a teacher of French and Spanish, he could no longer work. He took lessons in "cane travel" and, since he could still read if he had lots of light, he bought himself a floor lamp whose four bulbs together gave off 330 watts. In time that lamp would have a momentous effect on my life.

My son and I never used more than its top, 150 watt bulb. Soon we came to call it "Paul's lamp." He would sit under it by the hour when he wasn't playing his guitar or visiting with friends or volunteering at the church where we had met, answering the phone and fielding questions from visitors. We waited for the bleed into his "good eye" to be absorbed by surrounding tissues and hoped that somehow the series of specialists we went to would stave off any further hemorrhages. The doctors did their best. For a time his condition improved. But then came a second hemorrhage, then another and another. By 1981, Paul was totally blind.

Usually my husband made a fine show of keeping up his spirits but one day he came home seething with bitterness and resentment. Some stranger, seeing him with his cane and wanting to comfort him had told him, "Don't worry, someday you'll see again," meaning, of course, in the afterlife. "What a crock," my atheist husband roared to me, fury in his worn, once handsome face. "When it's over, it's over." Around New Year's Day, 1983, he came down with pneumonia. Three weeks later Paul passed on.

I never expected to sense him near me again. My 16-year-old son and I kept busy preparing for his memorial service and the open house we would hold that same day. For almost two weeks those duties kept us focused. The day after the memorial service—it was a Sunday—I felt lonely, let down. Somehow I would have to start rebuilding my life. Keith had a paper due the next day; I offered to type it for him and pressed him to put his draft into final form. We were standing in the living room of the Manhattan highrise apartment where the two of us had lived since 1969. Paul's lamp, unlit, was a few feet away. Suddenly *it turned itself on* and started flashing strangely, short flashes of light that came infrequently and seemingly in response to things we said.

At first it was incomprehensible. "That's weird," Keith said. We looked at each other, bemused. Nothing like this had ever happened since Paul bought that lamp several years before. And there was nothing wrong with the wiring in the building. And nothing else in the apartment seemed to be affected. The refrigerator still droned on; our hallway light glowed on, unchanging. Once more our eyes met—and suddenly Keith and I both understood. Paul was contacting us. How better could he let us know that now he could tell the difference between on and off, light and dark? The blind man we loved could see again!

We started laughing and crying and dancing around the lamp. Paul, who spoke French like a Frenchman, had lived in Paris for five happy years when he was young, had visited there often, had been the ultimate Francophile. "Now you can go see Paris again," Keith said and for a long moment the lamp blazed brighter.

Twice that evening, Paul's lamp came on by itself and flickered for a time mysteriously. Afterwards, returning to our accustomed skepticism, we checked its bulbs and switches and the outlet where it was plugged in. Nothing we found accounted for the way that it had behaved. My son—who in his senior year of high school would win two regional awards for scientific achievement—noted that it seemed to have difficulty flashing unless we were within about eight feet of it, and could not flash frequently or immediately in response. Keith theorized that Paul's spirit had only limited energy and capacity to respond. (Years later I would run across confirmation of this theory in a book by a distinguished British physicist, Sir Oliver Lodge, who in the early part of the 20th century wrote books on the paranormal. More about this in Chapter 9.)

The next day, I visited our church to pick up some phonograph records that had been played at Paul's memorial service. There I ran into Prabat, a Hindu friend of Paul's. Prabat was a thickset, warmhearted man in his fifties, trained as an engineer. As soon as he caught sight of me, his broad dark face lit up.

"I'm so glad to see you," he said, "I have something to tell you. Paul came to me in a dream. He took my hand. You know how he used to shake hands, very strong, very firm. I could *feel* him with my hand. He said he was happy now so I asked him to tell me more, to tell me where he was, what it had been like, you know, to die—but then he disappeared and the next thing ... I woke up."

Prabat laughed. "That dream was so real. I got out of bed and looked all over the house for him." That was when I told him what had happened with Paul's lamp.

"You mustn't worry," he said, "it's perfectly natural. For thirty days after someone dies, he can wander the earth at will."

He was speaking out of his Hindu tradition, happy to share it with me. So *that's* what Hindus believe, I thought. There are hundreds of millions of Hindus in the world, I figured, not to mention all the Buddhists who believe in reincarnation and the Chinese who practice ancestor worship, so they must believe in spirit survival too. Maybe, I decided, I'm not so crazy to believe that Paul's spirit may have survived.

I was struggling to keep my balance and deal with all my responsibilities. Inevitably, Paul's death had left me prone to tears and buffeted by waves of emotional turmoil. Somehow now, alone, I had to head a household with a teenage son and, if I was to pay the bills of that household, I'd have to go on running the architecture library at the City College of New York, something I'd been doing for the past seven years. Nonetheless, I was an Aquarian—notoriously adaptable—and a practiced writer and researcher. Prabat's experience and my own aroused my analytical side.

A couple of days after my conversation with Paul's Hindu friend, I scribbled down a log of strange things that had happened around the time of the memorial service. I headed it, "SUPER-NATURAL (?) EVENTS, WEEKEND OF FEBRUARY 6, 1983." At the time, I wasn't even familiar with the word "paranormal." Unlike "supernatural," which suggests that a phenomenon is magical or bizarre, "paranormal" suggests merely that science has not yet found a neat explanation for it. It never occurred to me then that anything more would happen to me, or to anyone else who had been close to Paul, that would suggest his spirit's presence on our plane. But lots more has. For 17 years I've kept up that log; now it's over 50 pages long.

A third of those pages cover events that happened that first year—but not all of these just happened to me. Many were perceived by Keith alone. With some irritation, my teenage son reported to me that Paul still seemed determined to parent him. Often when Keith should have been studying but instead was talking to a friend on the phone, a pin-up lamp in his room would flash. When it was time for him to go to bed, the lamp would turn off.

Twice, apparently paranormal incidents were noticed by me and another person who was in my company at the time—first a woman I worked with, later a male acquaintance. Jonathan, the office manager at our church and a friend of Paul's, reported other odd events to me. For years, as Paul coped with his growing blindness, he had helped out in the church office and brought along a portable radio to keep his mind occupied. After his death, a tiny earphone which Paul had used to listen to that radio kept turning up on Jon's desk there. "And sometimes," Jon told me, "I get this oddball sense I'm being *overheard.*"

None of us ever saw an apparition or heard Paul's voice. Instead, over half these apparently paranormal events involved electrical gadgets like lights, a fan, an air conditioner, a record player, two hairdryers and a hot pot. (Paul's lamp was most likely to flash when I was down in the dumps but was *not* thinking of him.) Other events involved the movements of small objects in symbolic or useful ways. For instance, one Friday afternoon when I'd forgotten to make an important phone call before the weekend, legal papers which had been thumbtacked for months onto a bulletin board in my bedroom fell down; they reminded me just in time to get in touch with my lawyer. No draft dislodged them and I didn't brush against them; I was several feet away when they rustled down onto my dresser.

Somehow Keith and I survived that first hard year without Paul. Then things started happening that recalled Paul's taste for puns. Keith went away to college. To liven up my empty nest, I invited two old friends over to dinner. Paul had known and liked both of them. The evening went well. After my guests left, I tidied up, then went to sleep. The next morning I found lying on the floor a small metal box of the herb, sage. Now, I hadn't used this herb the previous night, nor could it easily have fallen from the spice rack above. A wooden rod across the front of each shelf held its contents in place; nothing had ever fallen from this rack before. But sage had been Paul's favorite seasoning and in both French and English, "sage" has a complimentary meaning. This is especially true in French, Paul's second language, in which it can mean sensible and well-behaved as well as wise. Three years later, the can of sage again fell mysteriously. I had just generously tipped two of my building's maintenance men whom Paul had always liked and tipped similarly. Both times I could almost hear ghostly applause.

By now I was sensing paranormal contact far less often. Months, even years elapsed between shows of Paul's presence. During each long interval, I would assume that his spirit had moved on, that I would never sense him again. For me, the most striking evidence that I wasn't imagining things when I did indeed sense him is the gap in my log between July 10, 1990 and October 21, 1993. In 1991 I took early retirement from my job and moved from New York which had been my home for the past 24 years to Oregon where at first I knew almost no one. For over a year I suffered frequent bouts of loneliness. I would have welcomed a sense of Paul's presence but my log has no entries at all for that period. True, there was a light fixture in my kitchen which occasionally flickered but, because its flickering never seemed to correspond meaningfully with any thought or mood of mine, I never sensed anything paranormal to it. I wasn't the least bit surprised when in 1994, someone repainting my ceiling discovered that the fixture needed to be rewired.

By the fall of 1993 I was once again convinced that Paul would never communicate with me again. I was also becoming involved with Charles, the man who four years later would become my husband. When I invited three of Charles's relatives over for dinner, Paul's spirit popped by to give his blessing to my new beau.

Not long before my guests were due to arrive, I set to work to fix eggplant parmigiana while Charles, a helpful sort, started making a salad. Out of a kitchen drawer I pulled a grater and laid it down on a counter. It was a flat 11 x 5 inch stainless steel number with sharp-edged slots for shredding vegetables and such. I planned to use it to shred mozzarella; Charles planned to use it to grate a carrot for his salad. But for the moment neither of us was ready to use this common kitchen tool.

A few minutes later I was ready to shred my cheese—but that stainless steel grater was nowhere to be found. My new partner and I both looked high and low: on counters, in drawers, behind and under bags of produce. At last, we gave up in desperation. I sliced my cheese with a knife, Charles took a potato peeler to his carrot. Our guests arrived, we sat down to eat, then I got up to fetch dessert. And there on the counter where I'd left it in the first place was that runaway grater, like the prodigal son.

As I came back to the dinner table, Charles responded to the stunned expression on my face. "Is something wrong?" he asked me. I waved the grater at him and told him where I'd found it. As soon as we got over our astonishment, it was obvious to us both what Paul had meant to tell us: Charles was *greater*, far better for me, than any other man I'd ventured to date in the ten lean years since his death.

THINKING ABOUT SURVIVAL OF THE SPIRIT

I had quit my job and moved to Oregon to start a new life. I'd brought my log with me and lots of memories. For a long time I'd played with the idea of writing something about what I had experienced since Paul's death but one thing deterred me: dread of revisiting the pain of those last years with him. Throughout those years I had never stopped loving him—but that had only added to my suffering. Apprehension had become the fixed expression on my face. I lived in fear of each new hemorrhage and the damage it might do. I couldn't help sensing and sharing his anguish as, little by little, his sight was stolen from him.

At last, in the soft winter rains and bright, dry summers of the Willamette Valley, I healed. Paul's spirit had moved on, I knew. It was time I did the same. I started reading widely about the paranormal, particularly about survival of the spirit after death. As a professional librarian who had worked for years in a college library, I knew a great deal about research in many fields. Articles in scholarly journals were among the first things I checked.

Soon I ran across data on the multitude of people from different countries who had had experiences that resembled my own. For instance, when in their European Human Values Study, Gallup pollsters asked, "Have you ever felt that you were really in touch with someone who had died?" 33% of Italians said yes, as did 26% in Great Britain and West Germany. Icelanders topped the list with

41%. For Asians who, like my friend Prabat, took survival of the spirit for granted, the rate of contact experiences was *over twice as high.*

A study of mourning in Japan reported that 27 out of 30 Tokyo widows whose husbands had recently died in car accidents sensed their presence afterwards. Its author, a Japanese-American psychiatrist, pointed out that Japan's two religions, Buddhism and Shinto, both assume the presence of the deceased, at least at times. "According to traditional rites," he noted, "the spirits of the deceased can be called back to this world—usually by shamanistic rites similar to those widespread throughout Asia. . . . [If you were Japanese you would feel] in direct daily communication with your ancestors. The family altar would be your 'hot line.' . . . You could . . . ring the bell, light incense, and talk over the current crisis with one whom you have loved and cherished."

But even in Western cultures, responsible research by skilled professionals documented that healthy, normal individuals often sense apparent contact with the dead. Here, offered chronologically, are some tidbits I came up with:

- Interviews with 66 widowers and 227 widows in an area of Wales—almost all of those healthy enough to be interviewed—revealed that half the widowers and 46% of the widows had sensed some kind of after-death communication [ADC] with their departed mate. (Vivid dreams that seemed like visits from a loved one were not counted.) According to W. D. Rees, the general practitioner who reported this research in 1971, ADCs were usually perceived as helpful and pleasant. Those who had them were *not* particularly depressed or socially isolated. Instead, they were more likely to have had longer marriages, happier marriages, and marriages with children. Though ADCs were most likely to occur within the first year after a loved one's passing, sometimes they recurred for years, even decades. Often they continued after the widowed spouse remarried.

- A 1970s survey of residents of Los Angeles which drew samples from white, black, Japanese- and Mexican-American neighborhoods found that 44% of the 434 people interviewed thought they had had encounters with someone who was dead. Over a quarter of those who reported such an encounter said that the dead person actually visited or was seen at a seance.

- The ambitious Harvard Bereavement Study of widows and widowers from the Boston area followed scores of subjects for four years after they lost their mates. Three weeks after their loss, 44% of those who expressed a high degree of yearning for their dead spouse felt that "My husband/wife knows and sees everything I do." More surprising, almost a third of those in the "Low Yearning" category *also* agreed with this statement. Most of the widows sensed that their husband was with them some or all of the time. "One reported hearing her husband come to the door after work and put his key in the lock. Four others reported catching sight of their husband out of the corner of their eyes. In one case he was sitting in the living room ... in another he was standing by the door." The widows found this sense of presence comforting.

  Interviewed thirteen months after bereavement, almost half agreed with the statement that "I have a feeling that my husband watches over me." The researchers stressed that their subjects were *not* psychotic and, observed that since "bereaved people are often reluctant to reveal information ... that might be taken to indicate mental illness," these figures were probably an undercount.

- In 1982, an Arizona psychologist, David Balk, interviewed a sample of normal American teenagers who had lost a sister or brother. About half of them at times had thought they saw or heard their dead sibling. Several reported occurrences that they felt "involved actual contact with the sibling."

- In 1985, a team of Americans headed by P. Richard Olson, MD, studied 52 widowed people in a North Carolina nursing home, none of whom appeared to be mentally ill or confused. Over 60% of the 46 widows had sensed their husbands with them after death in some way. For almost all of them, the experience was a pleasant one. Two of the six widowers in the nursing home reported similar experiences.

Some of the most interesting data on American experiences of contact with the dead have been pulled together by Andrew M. Greeley, the distinguished sociologist, novelist and Catholic priest. Writing in 1989 he reported that in a poll conducted by the National Opinion Research Center (NORC), 42% of Americans said that at least once they'd felt that they "were really in touch with someone who had died." Impressed by the Olson study cited above, Greeley sorted through the data from that NORC poll to see how its *widowed* respondents had answered this question. "Of the 149 widowed," he reported, "129 were women and 20 were men. The proportion of widows reporting contact with the dead 'at least once or twice' was 64 percent."

Recently, a few researchers doing surveys of this kind have reassured their interview subjects that normal people often have "illusions or hallucinations" of loved ones who have passed on. Their rates of positive responses have gone through the roof.

- A 1993 study measured the feelings of 20 American university students, 18-27 years old, who had lost a parent at least two years before. The great majority of them agreed strongly with the statement, "I feel he/she is still with me at times."

- A 1993 Swedish study of 14 widowers and 36 widows in their seventies found that one month after bereavement, 89% of the women and 57% of the men reported some kind of after-death communication—this even though ADCs "are hardly recognized in Sweden. They are spoken about neither publicly nor among close friends." Only after these widows and widowers were told that such sensations were common did they "speak freely, expressing relief from thoughts that they 'might become or be considered insane.'" A year after bereavement, over half of them reported that they were still sensing contact with their lost mates.

- A 1995 study of Norwegian women, 44-79 years old, who had lost their husbands or live-in partners showed similar results. Soon after bereavement, almost three-quarters of them (29 out of 39) sometimes sensed their lost mate's presence. And a year later, *two-thirds* of them were still sensing ADCs.

Even more striking was an in-depth study by a Massachusetts psychologist, Dr. Roberta Dew Conant, of ten white middle-class, middle-aged homeowners who had recently lost their husbands. In Conant's opinion, all of them were adjusting well to their bereavement. Yet *every one of them* reported that, at least once, she had experienced "unbidden, consoling 'sense of presence' of the deceased." Their ADCs took many forms but most interesting to me for obvious reasons was the widow who reported that many important family events "were accompanied by flickering lights. The family 'came to believe' that dimming lights meant the deceased husband was communicating his presence."

Over the past few years, evidence for ADCs has mounted. In two scholarly yet eminently readable books, Louis E. LaGrand, Distinguished Service Professor Emeritus at the State University of New York, discusses after death contacts from the point of view of a certified grief counselor. In *Talking to Heaven,* a bestselling book by a well known medium, James Van Praagh lists "ways spirits let their loved ones know that they are around them *without* the use of a medium." Topping that list is lights, followed by other electrically operated devices. In *Hello from Heaven!,* Bill and Judy Guggenheim supply 353 thumbnail accounts of contact experiences culled from over 2,000 interviews. They document that spirits may come to us via many routes including dreams, the five senses and, yes, the meaningful misbehavior of electrical devices.

As my research on ADCs progressed, I decided to take a leap and do a series of interviews of my own. The prospect was tempting since I have a master's degree in sociology and have always found survey work fascinating. Besides, though I have the highest regard for the achievements of the Guggenheims and Prof. LaGrand, it is always useful in a field as new as this for independent researchers to replicate still controversial studies. My goal was not just to collect stories of spontaneous after-death contacts but to get a handle on who was most likely to experience them. Perhaps, I hoped, frequent perceivers of contact would open up to me, knowing that I myself had often sensed contact with a departed loved one.

Later I would discover that Father Greeley had called for interviews of just this sort. In 1975, drawing on a study of over 1,400 Americans done by NORC, he sketched out a profile of psychics, noting that people who grew up in a home where there was considerable tension were particularly likely to experience clairvoyance, telepathy and déjà vu. He also explored the phenomenon of contact with the dead. But lamenting the limitations of standard polling, he pointed out that, "We are badly handicapped by the fact that we were unable to ask our respondents any more than whether they had had such experiences. It would be important to know whether the experiences were dreaming or awake, whether there was conversation with the dead person [and] what the circumstances were at the time of contact. . . ."

Since the early 1990s when I started talking openly about my own paranormal experiences, I've discussed ADCs with hundreds who had experienced them firsthand. Since 1998, I've done 78 in-depth interviews with women and men who had had ADCs. All interviews were taped, transcribed, then analyzed. Twelve of my informants were personally known to my husband and/or me; several had been our friends for many years. The experiences they reported provided a standard of comparison for the stories of the others. As it turned out, there was no significant difference between the two groups of stories.

All but one of my informants gave every evidence of coping with their lives with at least average sanity and skill. They've told me not just about the ADCs they've had but far, far more. They've described their religious and spiritual backgrounds: what they were taught to believe and what they've come to believe as a result of spirit contacts. They've told me the context out of which their experiences flowed. They've entrusted me with secrets, some of which they had never shared before with another living soul. It has been humbling for me—yet enriching beyond measure. I have tried to keep faith with them, to mine wisdom out of their precious ore.

CONTACT EXPERIENCES AND THOSE WHO HAVE THEM

What constitutes a contact experience? The stereotypical contact, only too familiar to us from stage, screen and TV, is a visual one. Our trembling heroine sees a threatening ghost, our flabbergasted hero tries to deal with his late wife, glowing greenly and trailing filmy chiffon. Is this the way it really is? Well, not exactly.

Only one-eighth of the contact-with-the-dead experiences I collected involved sight at all. Some of these did indeed involve seeing a departed loved one, wholly or in part, clearly or hazily. But many other sight experiences involved seeing lights turn on or off or flicker at a particularly meaningful time, for no perceptible physical reason. (See Chapter 9 for more about these.) Still others involved the movement of an object, usually very small, associated with the lost person—a ribbon or a photo or a cherished tiny figurine. (Chapter 11 tells more about these.)

Three other senses—hearing, touch and smell—were mentioned about as frequently as sight but the most common vehicle for a contact experience was a vivid dream. Those who had ADCs in dreams reported that these dreams felt substantially different from the garden variety; many years later, they might remember them in loving detail. Sometimes their vivid dreams conveyed information they hadn't known before. More often the loved ones they perceived in dreams seemed to be visiting to reassure the dreamer that they were all right or to urge the dreamer to stop mourning and get on with his or her life. (Chapter 15 tells more about vivid, paranormal dreams.)

Almost as frequently, people perceived contact with the dead via telepathic communication, symbolic events, or that subtle awareness called "sense of presence." Telepathic communication, also called extra-sensory perception or ESP, is probably the best known of these three. (Though it generally involves communication between living persons it also occurs frequently between the dead and the living.) Many of the symbolic events reported to me involved extraordinary behavior by an animal or bird. Chapter 12 tells stories of a hummingbird and a fox, an owl, several beloved dogs and a wildly running horse, all of which conveyed information or comfort through their actions.

Clearly some people have many more ADCs than others. I myself was never aware of having any until I was in my forties; then I started having lots of them. Being widowed makes it a lot more likely that you'll have contact experiences. But a number of the people I interviewed, over two-thirds of whom had never been widowed, had had five or more ADCs; often they started having them early in life. It's fair to call these people "sensitives." In many another culture, given their ability to receive messages from the spirit world, they might be groomed to be shamans or mediums. What gave them their special powers? In Chapter 16, I offer evidence from a number of scholarly studies that certain kinds of childhood experiences tend to create sensitives.

Only too many people in our society believe that all talk of contact with spirits is just so much wish fulfillment and woowoo fantasy. I, too, was brought up to think this way. In the university settings where I earned three degrees, denial of anything that implied that there might be spiritual forces afoot in the world seemed to be an article of faith. Yes, an article of *faith*. Like Madonna, we were all supposed to be material—and materialistic—girls and boys focused on making our mark in the one short life we had.

Now skepticism may well be a healthy stance from which to view many intellectual issues—but only if the skeptic is open-minded enough to take in all the evidence and move on accordingly. Unfortunately, only too often we run into close-minded, compulsive disbelievers determined not to acknowledge the conclusions argued by the facts. For them, denial of anything resembling an afterlife seems to be a kneejerk reaction. Such readers probably abandoned this book several pages ago. But for those whose minds are open, I offer the next two chapters. Both of them, I think, offer irrefutable evidence for the survival of the human spirit after death.

2

Sensing Someone Else's Death

THERE'S MORE TRUTH THAN POETRY tucked into this nineteenth century song:

> My grandfather's clock was too large for the shelf
> > So it stood ninety years on the floor.
> It was taller by half than the old man himself
> > Though it weighed not a pennyweight more.
> It was bought on the morn of the day that he was born,
> > And was always his treasure and pride
> *But it stopped short, never to go again,*
> > *When the old man died.*
>
> *Ninety years without slumbering (tick, tock, tick, tock)*
> *His life-seconds numbering, (tick, tock, tick, tock)*
> *It stopped short, never to go again,*
> > *When the old man died.*

In a bygone era, vaudevillians warmed the hearts of audiences with this sentimental ballad. Families gathered around the piano in the parlor to sing it together. It rang true to them because its last line was part of American folklore, telling of a clock that stopped mysteriously, of its own accord, when its owner died.

16

It's still happening. Here is what three of my interviewees told me. First, from Charlie, a 55 year-old college professor:

> Right after my dad died, I noticed that there were about three clocks whose batteries went out. I mean you could say, "Of course, the battery died," but it just coincidentally happened right around that time. Now when the clocks went out, there were also problems with both of the TVs. On one of them it was the remote. On the other one, it was something about the channel changer. So all those things went wrong at about the same time. And I thought, just statistically, that seems unlikely.

Phyllis, a 49 year-old registered nurse, told me about something that happened when her father-in-law died.

> My father-in-law had been in the hospital about five days, he'd had surgery. All his kids except my husband were there and they told us later that at the time their dad passed away, when they went back home they found in his workshop that the clock had stopped. It had stopped at the time he died. And they're not a family that believe any of that stuff. So they just thought it was odd.

Colleen, 52, is a former real estate broker. Here's what happened at her brother's home after their father died:

> My brother has two big, wind-up antique clocks. I mean, these are huge and both of these clocks stopped at the very same time. My dad made his transition in his sleep. They found him at like five something in the morning and the clocks both shut down a little after two so that's probably when he passed on.

From 1935 on, the Parapsychology Laboratory at Duke University was noted for doing experiments on-site to test the reality of extra-sensory perception. In 1948, they started collecting accounts of spontaneous events—things that "just happened"—which seemed to involve the paranormal. Everyday people who had heard of the lab mailed in letters describing unusual experiences they had

had. Most of these involved ESP. But in 1963, Louisa Rhine—one of the laboratory's founding scientists—reported on the 178 cases in the Duke collection which involved what she called "spontaneous physical effects" or psychokinesis.

These events involved physical objects which seemed to act by themselves—and in ways that might give clues to something that was happening at a distance. "An example," she said, "would be a case in which a clock stops or a picture falls" at a time when a loved one dies faraway. In 37 of the cases she reported, a clock stopped or started around the time when someone who meant a lot to the perceiver was dying. Most of these, like the grandfather's clock in the song, had to be wound by hand. Sometimes two or three clocks stopped at one time. A woman in Florida reported:

> We had a pendulum clock which we wound every Sunday . . . a musical clock which we wound every evening and . . . my husband's pocket watch. On the evening before Thanksgiving day, 1913 . . . all three clocks stopped at once. My husband . . . gave the weights a shove, shook the little musical clock and his pocket watch; and they ran again. In two weeks we [learned] that my husband's father in Austria had died the same day and hour.

The odds are astronomical against three clocks in one household stopping at the same, deeply meaningful time. But since these events were said to have happened at least 35 years before that woman in Florida reported them, it's easy to speculate about the fuzziness of her memory. The wife of an Air Force pilot told a more contemporary story about an event that had happened the previous year. Right before it occurred, she sensed impending disaster.

> The noon my husband left I said, "Be careful and take care of yourself,"—a thing which I had never done before as it was against the rules for a brave Air Force wife. Later in the afternoon I took a nap and at 3:26 awoke like a shot. . . . The clock had stopped and two hours later I was informed that my husband had crashed and died around 3:30.

Phenomena like these are called death coincidences (DCs). Here "coincidence" means that two events coincided; it doesn't imply that this happened by chance. DCs don't have to involve clocks. Or premonitions. Though sometimes they do. People who are open to paranormal messages can receive information in many different ways.

In Scotland, a form of sensitivity called second sight is common, especially in the Western Isles and the Highlands. People gifted with this power have visions spontaneously while awake that give information about something distant in time or space. Sometimes they enable the psychic to predict something happy, like what fine young Scotsman a blushing young thing will marry. More commonly the perceiver learns what person in the village is fated to die next or senses a distant person's death at the time when it occurs.

Twenty-three of my interviewees reported extraordinary experiences that came to them around the time when someone who mattered a lot to them died. Here are some of their stories. In the first three, the perceivers saw visions or apparitions.

Beverly, 42, is an administrative assistant for a non-profit group.

> When I was 7 years old, I was lying in bed and I *saw* my Aunt Ruby and she said to me, "Don't worry, child, everything will be all right," and I felt a brush near my shoulder. When I ran down the hall to tell my mom and dad that I'd just seen my Aunt Ruby, somebody called and said she had died. The phone call came as I was running down the hallway. My father was listening to my mom screaming and listening to me at the same time and so he shouted and pointed at me, "Go back to your own room." And so we never talked about it again.

Beverly was the first person I interviewed for my survey and many of the things she had to say turned out to be classic. Most striking to me was the way her father turned a deaf ear to her remarkable perception. In later interviews I would hear similar stories. Again and again, families shortchanged themselves of comforting messages because they didn't dare acknowledge the reality of after-death communication. And sensitive youngsters soon learned the hard lesson that they'd better not tell others about what they perceived through some paranormal sense.

Katya, 58, is in the real estate business. She told of a healing contact experience she had when she was a young mother. Her Uncle Ted had doted on her first child but when she and her husband adopted an African-American child—Katya and her husband were white—his reaction was totally different.

My husband and I had our first daughter, Lee Ann, and Uncle Ted was very much a part of Lee Ann's birth and celebration. Then later we adopted Lisette when she was six days old so we called my uncle and told him we were coming to introduce Lisette to him. We dressed her up in a little white dress with a white bonnet and white shoes. We were so excited! We met him in a hotel he owned—and my uncle completely ignored Lisette and ran after Lee Ann who was a toddler and I kept holding Lisette up to him and he would turn the other way. It was awful, very hurtful, because I had been close to my uncle and never thought there'd be any difficulty. He was the last person in the world that I felt would not accept this racial integration. All the other members of our family had.

So I wrote him and told him I was hurt and that I hoped he would come to enjoy and love the little person that we loved. He was ill at this time. I never heard from him and I don't know how short a time it was after the letter writing, but I woke up one morning and I told my husband that I'd had a vision of Uncle Ted. He was in our dining room over near where our birdcage was and he was standing there in his black slacks, his white shirt and his red sweater and he had his arms outstretched and I went, "Uncle Ted," and I ran to hug him and he said, "No, don't touch me. I just came to tell you that I love *all* of you very, very much." I think this was after I woke up, I'm not sure. And I told my husband and he exclaimed, "Wow," and the phone rang and it was my brother and he said, "Uncle Ted died."

The experience was such a love experience for me that I no longer was in doubt. There was just such joy and reconciliation. At the funeral, I told my dad, who's a Presbyterian minister, and his two sisters and their mouths dropped. They never validated me or dismissed me, either way. First I was worried about speaking out of turn and then I finally decided I had had to tell them how I felt about Uncle Ted. But it was never talked about again.

R.J., a 57 year-old man, is a retired health professional who has lived happily with another man for many years. Openly gay and proud, he reported two death coincidences.

> I had a friend in Hawaii who was dying of AIDS who I had mentored for a couple of years. I was down at the beach on a Sunday morning. I'm sitting there talking to some people and I look over and I say, "My god, I thought Laurie was in the hospital." Now here he is sitting with two other people that I had never seen before. They were surrounded by the most incredible white glimmering kind of light. It didn't look like a sunlight thing. It was like a halogen light looks. I looked at my watch and the next day I found out that was exactly the time he died.
>
> Another time, we're sitting on the beach and I said, "My god, look at that. There's David out there backstroking," and Will, my friend, said, "Oh, my god." I said, "Let's check the time." And David, the person who was passing away at the time, was just on the Big Island—which is not more than a hundred miles away—but now he doesn't swim and he certainly doesn't do the backstroke but that was exactly the time he passed away.

Two accounts come from a mother and daughter whom I interviewed together. Sharon, 54, the mother, is a school custodial aide who has a clairvoyant's knack for finding lost things. An intensely religious Methodist, she credits most of her paranormal knowledge to divine assistance. This is what she sensed when her own mother was dying.

> The day my mom passed, I knew she was sick, I knew she was in the hospital and so I was praying for her, and my bedroom became so dark as if death itself was at the doorstep, and I got up, went down and told my husband, "Mom just passed away." This was at 9 o'clock in the morning. And my husband says, "No, don't accept it, don't believe it." So 3 o'clock my brother called. I says, "Butch, sit down, I want to talk to you." He said okay, and so I said, "Mom passed away at 9 o'clock this morning." He goes, "How'd *you* know?" I said, "I wasn't there but the Lord told me this, 'Quit praying, don't pray no more.'"

Sharon's story bears a striking resemblance to a traditional tale recounted by Martin Buber. It was first told by Eastern European hasidic Jews about a *tzaddik,* a particularly holy man, who sensed the passing of a beloved friend.

> The hour Rabbi Levi Yitzhak died, a *tzaddik* teaching in a distant city suddenly interrupted his discourse . . . and said to his disciples: "I cannot go on. Everything went dark before my eyes. The gates of prayer are closing. Something must have happened to the great worshiper, to Rabbi Levi Yitzhak."

One of my interviewees supplied me with a written account that also resembles Sharon's story:

> The night my uncle Ed died in World War II, my grandmother was sitting in the living room when she saw a black cloud obscure the light shining in the kitchen. She turned to my grandfather and announced that Ed was dead. News came from Washington several days later confirming her announcement.

Sharon's daughter, a 31-year-old social worker, offered the following death coincidence which involved just that subtle perception which researchers call sense of presence.

> My father had been ill, he had a bad heart. So I was home, I was living about an hour and a half from where my family was at that time, and I can remember laying on the floor, watching some TV and feeling his presence. It was probably like 11:30, 11:45 at night, and just feeling his closeness and I knew. And my mother called me the next day and said that he had died during the night. When he passed, I believe, is when he came to me.

Carol, 40, is a graduate student in environmental science. Gifted with a psychic's sensitivity, she detected meaning in seemingly commonplace events.

> My stepmother was a lovely, lovely woman. She got pancreatic cancer and died nine months after it was diagnosed. The night that

she died, it was around 10:15 and I was in my bedroom in Victoria [British Columbia]. All of a sudden there was like a knock on the wall. I turned around and the curtains were blowing in my window but there was no breeze outside. I just knew that was her and I knew she must've died because there was no one there knocking on the wall and there wasn't any breeze. I didn't get the phone call till 5 or 6:30 the next morning. My sister was crying. She said Hannah had died in Bethlehem, Pennsylvania at 1:15 in the morning. So that was 10:15 at night in Victoria. I felt really sad 'cause she had died. I felt happy that she came to see me, like to let me know.

This experience reported by Mary-Minn, 43, an editor, involved only hearing.

I was very close to my grandfather. He had a wonderful sense of humor and he always related to me as though I were a little kid. And he'd tease me. He'd say very affectionately in this real deep voice, "Mary-Minn, you're a baddie, a real baddie." He said that from the time I was about four or five and he still said it when I was in my twenties. Well, he went into a coma for a week or two. I wasn't talking to most people in my family—we had had some horrible feud. But I'd been keeping up with my grandmother and I knew he was in a coma and would probably die. So I was sitting in my office one rainy afternoon, typing up a disbursement voucher, and suddenly this deep voice came out and said, "Mary-Minn, you're a baddie, a real baddie." And that was it. I knew it was him and I knew that nobody else heard it. I mean I knew that he had just died, he had just expired. Well, the phone rang about two minutes later and he had.

The next two accounts involve feelings of grief that at first seemed mysterious, uncalled for. This story comes from Bob, 59, an engineer.

On the night of Mother's Day, I broke out into sobbing. It started in bed and then sitting on the bed, and then leaning my head in the sink and Boom! Like torrents. Men don't talk about crying a lot and I don't normally cry, period. But this was something that happened and I didn't know what to make of it and then the next morning we got the word that my father had died that night. I don't know what it means, I just know those two facts occurred. It certainly seemed like more than just happenstance.

Anna, 52, a social worker, had a similar experience.

> I was visiting my daughter. It should have been a happy time but for about three days I kept crying. I was so sad and I had no idea why I was so sad. But I just kept being overwhelmed with these feelings of loss. And when I got back home, I learned that a very dear former mentor of mine had died. So the day before he died and for a couple days after, I was grieving the loss of my teacher. You might call him my ideal father. So I didn't know what had happened to him but I was so sad.

The death coincidence experienced by John, 65, a retired journalist and photographer, also involved a beloved adviser and guide but it entailed more joy than sorrow.

> My wife and I were walking along and I had an overpowering feeling of the presence of this man, Harper B., who had been my mentor for maybe ten years, a very spiritual and knowledgeable person. I didn't see him. It was dark, about 8 or 9 o'clock at night. He lived in California which was hundreds of miles away. Now, Harper was not ill. I was not concerned about him at all. This just came out of the blue. I stopped in my tracks and said, "Harper!" I was just filled with the sense of him. It was a feeling of intense euphoria, like he was within me or we were one. I was overwhelmed by his presence and it was all positive. Then I talked to my wife about him a little bit and we finished our walk and got home. And the next morning a call came that he had died the night before.

In the following three cases, women learned through dreams that other women they'd been close to had died and now were happy.

Cindy, 42, runs a small business. Her mother was one of the first people in the United States to be diagnosed with mad cow disease. Cindy's father was taking care of her. Since no one knew how much longer her mother might live, Cindy met with family members to discuss what should be done.

My father couldn't go on for another ten years taking care of her. That night I had this just incredibly strong dream. My mom came to me. Now she had really thin hair so she'd worn wigs ever since I was a kid. And she came to me in a dream and she didn't have her wig on, and she just said, "Time for me to go." Very calmly. "I can't stay any longer and it's just time." And she turned and she went to like a staircase and she went up, and the next thing I saw is like a really green lawn that goes up a hill and she was sitting on a stone bench there and she said, "I'm fine." And then my dad called at 6 o'clock that morning and said she'd passed away. I didn't find out until three or four months later that my brother had had the same dream. We were talking and I said, "You know, I had this really strange dream," and I told him about it and he said, "Oh, my god. I had just about the same thing."

Summer, 53, is a dancer and dance ethnologist who has taught at the college level. Her mother, who had been a first grade teacher for thirty years and was greatly loved in the community, died at 58, when Summer was in her twenties. For years Summer had troubling dreams which suggested to her that her mother's spirit was "kind of lost. I'm not sure she knew she was dead in the beginning. Like she would come back and sneak around and look around the corner at us. And she was alone and I'd try to bring her into the living room and she would start crying and say no. We were worried about her being in pain and we couldn't help her, her being lonely. We couldn't reach her so I gave up on dreams, I didn't want to dream anymore." Meanwhile her mother's mother lived on to be 92, at which time she still appeared to be in good health.

Then I had what was the strongest, most vivid dream of my life. All of a sudden I was transported to our old family home and then in comes my grandmother and in comes my mother and it was as real to me then as we are sitting here talking. And we hugged and kissed and laughed and giggled and we were just talking away and then I said, "Wait, what are we doing here?" And I realized my mother had been dead for 10 years. I didn't think my grandmother was dead.

Well, they smiled at me. We were sitting at the kitchen table. And they said, "We don't want you to worry and we're all right. We're home, everything's fine and we'll see you again soon." And then it was gone and I woke up. I mean, it was in technicolor and everything. And I woke up my partner and I told him all about it, and it was like two or three in the morning and I took note of the time. Next morning my dad woke us up with a call and he said, "Grandma died last night," and he said when she'd died, and it was within minutes of the time that I noted.

Elizabeth, 64, is a hairdresser who emigrated from Hungary with her husband, a movie cameraman. While she was living in California as a young married woman with two tiny children, her landlady, Hazel, befriended her and helped her learn English. After Elizabeth and her family moved away, the two women kept in touch. Then Hazel had a stroke.

One evening I went to bed and had a dream that I was standing at the foot of Hazel's hospital bed and Hazel was just lying there peacefully. And suddenly she sat up—but her body was still on the bed lying down. Some part of her sat up in a flowing motion, sitting up and standing up and lifting, elevating toward the ceiling. She was in white and she had white hair and she had this unbelievably, totally giving, loving, sweet, happy smile on her face as she was looking down at me, and as she was lifting toward the ceiling and disappeared into the ceiling. I woke up, I looked at the clock. It was 11:38 p.m. Next day her husband called me and said Hazel passed away at 11:38 p.m.

Phyllis, the registered nurse quoted early in this chapter, sensed something in her own body which identified a dying loved one to her.

I had a great-uncle who was like a grandfather to me. Very close. And he had Parkinson's disease. His hand trembled. He had been hospitalized and he was very ill. Well, I'd been working full time and I was taking a 15 minute break in the lunchroom and I had my feet up. I got into a space where I was very, very relaxed and my hands were in the pockets of my jacket. And suddenly one of my hands started to tremble. And I suddenly got upset without realizing. I started to cry a little. So I kind of glanced at the time and it was a little after two in the afternoon and I thought what could this possibly be?

I came home that evening—I was living with my parents at the time—and there were some cars in front of the house. And I went up to the front door and I remember someone opening the door and telling me my great-uncle had died. And I asked what time it happened and it happened at around that time.

Like Phyllis, most of the people I interviewed had had more than one "psi" experience. [The word "psi" covers a broad range of paranormal phenomena including telepathy, after-death communication, precognition, clairvoyance and psychokinesis.] Several times in their life, the average interviewee had sensed something meaningful that came, apparently, through a non-physical route— or at least via a path that physics has not as yet identified. Often these involved ESP contacts with the living, not after-death contacts.

The typical volunteer reported 3-5 experiences, though a few said they'd had only one and others mentioned having dozens, even countless experiences. Maxine had had dreams of a dead child several nights a week for a year, Connie had received helpful telepathic messages that came, when needed, many times a year over decades. Jerry had telepathic conversations almost nightly for 4 or 5 years with his dead wife; they guided him as he raised their kids till they came of age. (More about Connie and Jerry in Chapter 3; more about Maxine in Chapter 8.) Still, for the great majority of the people I interviewed, psi experiences of contact with the dead were infrequent.

Nonetheless, over one-fifth of these sensitives reported having the convincing death coincidences recounted in this chapter— sensations of contact that came to them within the 24 hour period that bracketed a loved one's death. Compulsive disbelievers like to attribute to chance anything that people learn through paranormal means. The odds are absurdly high against death coincidences like these being accidental.

Will your unique personality or mine survive after death in some spirit form? And if a spirit can survive, can it communicate with those it left behind? These are hardly new issues. In the 1880s, a number of outstanding English intellectuals, including leading scientists, came together to search for the answers to questions like these. They formed the Society for Psychical Research (SPR), which still is going strong and is based in London. Soon they attracted distinguished members from abroad as well.

The honor roll of the SPR's past presidents includes the American psychologist William James, the Nobel Prize-winning French physiologist Charles Richet, as well as British Prime Minister A. J. Balfour, not to mention numerous eminent physicists and philosophers, plus scholars drawn from other disciplines. Probably the society's most famous member was Sir Arthur Conan Doyle, the creator of Sherlock Holmes. Early on, the SPR took a special interest in death coincidences because it was possible—using objective, mathematical means—to gauge whether reports of them might simply be due to chance.

First they did a three-year study of what they called "spontaneous hallucinations of the sane." Over 400 volunteer interviewers asked 17,000 people if, when awake, they had ever "had a vivid impression of seeing or being touched by a living being or inanimate object, or of hearing a voice; which impression [apparently] was not due to any external physical cause." Those who answered yes—over 13% of those questioned—were then asked to answer a short list of questions about what they had sensed. Most of them, perhaps afraid of seeming demented, acknowledged having had only one such experience.

The data collected in this Census of Hallucinations, reported over a hundred years ago in 1894, provided a wealth of evidence both for spontaneous ESP contacts between living persons and for after-death contacts. Still the SPR's researchers were only too aware that skeptics might ask: Was there any significant basis for the perceptions people *thought* they had? Death coincidences, these researchers judged, were a special case since it was easy to pinpoint the particular date when the person who was sensed had died.

Had people just imagined lots of psychic contacts and had many of these contacts just accidentally occurred around the time of the other person's death? Of the almost 1,300 psi experiences that had been reported in the Census, 299 involved some sort of contact with the dead—and over a quarter of these contacts occurred within 12 hours of the death of the other person. "The fact that each of us only dies once," the SPR's analysts observed dryly, "enables us to calculate . . . the probability that that death will coincide with any other given event"—namely, a psychic perception of the dying person by someone else who was nowhere nearby.

The society's scrupulous researchers leaned over backward to be conservative in their count of death coincidences. For instance, they dropped from their count 8 which had been experienced before the age of 10, and 7 which had been reported by people who had also had other psi experiences—including telepathic contacts with the living—even though they asserted their belief that such perceivers might be accurate and reliable. Pruning their data in this way, they eventually slashed their count of death coincidences from 80 to 30. Then they weighed those 30 events against the probability that any given psi perception would involve a person dying on that day.

They attacked this problem in two different ways. Each time they came out with odds of over 400 to 1. Had they used that original tally of 80 rather than 30 as their count of death coincidences, the odds would have exceeded 1,000 to 1. Armed with these numbers, the SPR's researchers concluded that "Between deaths and [psi contacts with] a dying person a connexion exists which is not due to chance." What they had proven to the satisfaction of any reasonable person was that around the time of death, some aspect of the dying person was likely to communicate in paranormal fashion with the living. And neither walls nor distance were obstacles to the spirit.

Returning to the specific death coincidences reported in this chapter, we find even more striking evidence of the reality of psi contact at the time of death, the *specific* time of death. In nine of the cases reported in this chapter, a paranormal event occurred within *minutes* of the death of a loved one. These include one story from the files of Louisa Rhine, Phyllis's account about her father-in-law's clock, and the personal experiences of Beverly, Katya, R.J.,

Sharon, Carol, Mary-Minn and Elizabeth—not to mention the song about the grandfather's clock! Leaning over backwards to be conservative in our calculations, let's say that these events occurred within a 20 minute window: 10 minutes on either side of the time of death. Such a 20-minute segment is just 1/72nd of a day. What might the odds be against "coincidences" like these occurring by chance?

Over the years, compulsive disbelievers have tried to characterize such communications at the time of death as ESP experiences which prove nothing about the *survival* of the spirit *after* death. (Of course, when dealing with other cases, these skeptics are likely to pooh-pooh extra-sensory perception as well!) In the next chapter we'll look at other contemporary cases which should prove to any reasonable person that the spirit can indeed survive.

3

Knowledge and Guidance from the Other Side

IN ALL OF THE CASES DESCRIBED IN THIS CHAPTER, people received valuable information which they believe came from spirit sources. In most of these cases, there seems to be nowhere else from which it could have come.

Tom, 57, is a compactly built, confident man who has worked for many years as a manager in the wood products industry. Two months before I interviewed him, his second wife, Norma, died under circumstances that at first were mysterious. Late on a Thursday night she started out alone, driving their pickup a couple of hundred miles north from Oregon, their home state, to the house where they'd been living for the past few years in Washington State. For days Tom kept trying to phone her there. When she never answered, he went back to the place himself and discovered that Norma had never reached there. He checked her credit cards and discovered that at 3:15 Friday morning she'd bought gas about 65 miles south of their Washington home. Now he started trying to follow her likely route, on a major highway that cuts through sometimes rugged terrain, looking for her pickup along the road. On Tuesday, when he still couldn't find her, he reported her as missing to the sheriff's department. They started an intensive search by plane through all the canyons along the route but at first they didn't find anything. This is how Tom described what happened next.

I had really been stressed, hadn't slept and you're tied up in knots because you're thinking of the worst possible things that could happen to someone and it just tears you up inside. But between 4:30 and 5:30 that afternoon, I got this sense of peace. I had a cell phone with me so I called her daughter and I told her, "I don't know what's going on but I know we're gonna find your mom, I just feel really good." And she said she felt the same way, "I feel good all of a sudden."

So I'm driving to the town where I grew up and I've driven this road a thousand times so you just kind of drive on automatic, you know where everything is. So I got into this little trance—and I *heard* her. She said, "Honey, honey." I said, "Where are you, Norma?" Of course I'm thinking this in my head, I didn't *hear* her voice but I knew it was her. She said, "Come and find me. It's cold here. There's nobody here and I'm lonesome."

I said, "Well, where are you?" she said, "I don't know. I can hear the cars going by but nobody stops. I can see the sun shining through the trees but I don't really know where I'm at...."

Well, between 4:30 and 5:30 the sun sets in the west so I'm thinking that she's on the west side of a hill and the sun's filtering through the trees and the reason the plane didn't see her is that she's under heavy foliage. "My head hurts," she says, "it really hurts. I can move my left arm but I can't move my right arm, I don't know what's wrong with it. I can't feel my legs, I think they're broken. Come and find me. I love you."

"I love you too," I said, "just you hang in there." And I'm thinking that she's talking to me so she's okay. We're gonna find her, she's gonna make it. So I immediately called her daughter and I told her, "I think I just talked to your mother. She said her head hurts, she's close to the highway. She can't use her right arm, she can't feel her legs, and I think she's on the west side because she can see the sun shining through the trees."

That evening the sheriff's office called and said that they'd found my pickup and they'd found her and she was dead but the details were sketchy coming in. Later that evening the sheriff called and said the pickup was totally destroyed and they'd found Norma about a hundred feet *below* the pickup. She'd taken the windshield out with her—she wasn't wearing a safety belt—and by his observation, he said, she'd died instantly.

Then I waited for the phone call from the coroner's office. Well, the coroner was a lady, one of the nicest people. She told me about the details because she had to go up and pronounce the body dead, and I said, "Can you describe anything about the body from what you could observe?" And she said that Norma had severe head lacerations, bruising on the right side of her head because she took the full impact of the windshield. Her right arm had a severe compound fracture. So I said, "What about her legs?" "Well," she said, "her back was broken so she wouldn't be able to feel her legs." I had told her what I thought I had perceived and she said that she has been on similar bad accidents like this and people had had somewhat similar experiences and she said, "I *believe* that, I believe that you *did* talk to your wife."

Probably I should have checked Tom's story with the coroner's office soon after I heard it but I was busy doing other interviews and Tom was busy rebuilding his life, dealing with his grief while he found a new place to live and, eventually, a new job in Oregon. In fact, it was months before I talked to Tom again. He told me in what county his wife's accident had taken place and the name of the woman, whom I'll call here Carlotta, that he thought was coroner there. When I phoned the coroner's office, Carlotta answered the phone.

She was the chief deputy coroner, she told me, and she remembered the case well, called Tom by name and confirmed that his wife, Norma, had died in a motor vehicle accident in May 1998. Unfortunately she couldn't confirm the details of Norma's injuries; they were sealed by the court. To hear them from her, I'd have to subpoena her. "But I can tell you something else," she said. "I do know there was a psychic involved. There was a lady from the east end of the county that found her, that sent us to where she was. She didn't give anybody her name." When I relayed this information to Tom, he was surprised at first—but then it made sense to him. "My wife must've been broadcasting," he said, "she must've been reaching out all over the place. When she got through to that psychic, whoever that lady was, that must've been when Norma's daughter and I got that feeling of peace."

Tom's story, touching as it may be, has one especially curious aspect: the contrast between what he sensed paranormally and what he missed. Tom clearly identified his wife's injuries as she might have perceived them—yet he never picked up the crucial fact that she was dead. To a serious student of psi this is hardly surprising. Gaps like Tom's in paranormal messages crop up all the time. This is probably a major reason why, once the scientific method came into favor, it so thoroughly displaced psychic techniques for obtaining information.

Unlike a mathematical formula or a chemical reaction which, once identified, yields the same results again and again, the news that comes to minds in trance or meditation is likely to be hazy and incomplete. This contrast fuels the prejudice held by many scientists that all revealed truth is hardly worthy of mention, perhaps beneath contempt. Nonetheless, left brain thinking can have its own shortcomings. In Tom's case, the sheriff's search by plane over a heavily wooded area failed to find his wife's body until a psychic called to give them guidance. Apparently there's plenty of value in right brain "intuition," whatever its ultimate source may be.

Paula, 67, looks at least ten years younger than her calendar age. Brought up with no interest or belief in the paranormal, she holds a Ph.D. in psychology and has taught on the graduate level. Eight years before I interviewed her, she received technical information from the other side that could not conceivably have come from anywhere else. Twelve years earlier, in 1980, a series of events involving her late husband first alerted her to the possibilities of psi.

> I'm gonna go back to before Alain died. He went through a long illness with lung cancer. During the last few weeks he had an experience in which he was sitting on the couch and dozed off and it seemed to me that he stopped breathing. I thought he was gone. Then he took another breath, opened his eyes, and he said, "I had to tell you this." And he related what has now come to be known as a rather classic near death experience. At the end of the tunnel, standing in the light he saw his sister and his mother, both of whom were long gone. They were beckoning to him and he said, "It felt so

welcoming and so warm. I wanted to join them, I wanted out of this misery. And I was going toward them and I stopped and thought, no, I have to tell Paula about this. I pulled myself back and I am here to tell you that I now understand that I will be able to watch over you. I will be able to protect you and lead you forward."

Then he said something that turned out to be very interesting. He said, "A lot of the men we know are going to hit on you." And he proceeded to name five or six people who are dear friends, some of whom I would've thought might make a move and some of whom I would never have thought would make a move. And he said, "These are not the right people. I will help find the person that I want you to remarry."

Now Alain was a physicist whose specialty was theoretical physics, mathematical physics. He was not a spiritual person. He was not a religious person. Things like that were not high on his list. He was somebody who had grown up in the French rational educational system and anything that was a rational expression, he understood. He was not a touchy-feely person. So from *him*, this was very surprising.

So another six weeks go by and Alain does die and life is moving on. About a year and a half later, I'm reflecting on this and one by one, the men who he had named, both married and unmarried had made their move. And each time it happened, I would sort of chuckle to myself and say, "You're not the guy, pal!" *[Laughs]* Because I knew. I just knew.

Well, time goes by, two years, and I'm thinking, I can't do the singles scene. I can't do the meat market. Then playing tennis one day I meet a very interesting man and we have dinner together. We're sitting having dinner and he begins to tell me jokes because sometimes men, to cover their own discomfort, will relate to people by telling jokes. Well, one after the other he is telling stories that Alain would tell until I would kick him under the table because all our friends had heard them before. One joke after another. And I'm thinking, this is weird. This is really weird. Then he tells me about his college fraternity and it turns out he had been a member of the same fraternity that Alain was, only at a different college. And I thought, I better pay attention here. I think I'm getting a message. Well, to shorten that story, two years later he and I were married and this is my current husband. And he often will say that he blesses Alain's memory because Alain brought him to me.

All this is preface to an even more uncanny story. Paula had a brilliant son whom we'll call Ari. Among other things, he was a whiz at computers. When Ari was 30, he died suddenly of a chronic disease that is rarely fatal. At first his mother was almost inconsolable. A year to the day after his passing, she moved into her summer home. She was trying to assemble the components of a computer system that had been disassembled the previous fall so it could be stored elsewhere.

> I revved up the computer and I was ready to put it all together but I got these crazy error messages, nothing was working. It was working enough so that I could get DOS error messages but nothing would come up on the screen, just garbage. That evening I gave up in despair. I lit a memorial candle for Ari and spoke to Ari a little bit, looked at some of the photographs, and I went to sleep. Woke up at two in the morning and I heard a voice say, "Go to the computer and I'll tell you what to do."

> I sat down. My husband is asleep in the bedroom and the computer is in the bedroom but I turned it on and I'm sitting there in front of the screen and I am typing strings of computer commands in a language I don't know. Because I don't know computer language. I have never programmed, *never*, but I'm typing these strings of commands that have symbols and letters and numbers. This goes on for about 45 minutes, strings and strings and strings of it. And then I hit ENTER and everything works. And I understood that Ari was there to talk me through this. And when I was finished and everything was working—it was now 3:30 or 4 in the morning—I went back to sleep and I slept very soundly, and in my sleep I heard Ari's voice say, "Now mom, you can't count on me doing this all the time." And he said this in a way that only a 30 year old son would say this to a mother, namely, "Come on now, get yourself together and learn how to do some of these things yourself."

Connie, 62, is a cheerful, articulate woman with sparkling brown eyes and a warm, capable manner. For 20 years, until she took early retirement, she was personnel administrator at a major hospital. She attributes much of her competence on that job to help from the spirits of loved ones who'd passed on.

When she was a child, her home situation was highly stressful. The nearby home of her grandmother and her uncle was a refuge for her.

> My grandmother never had an unkind word about anybody or anything. I never knew her to get really agitated. She was always a very kind, soft-spoken woman. My uncle was pretty much the same way. My uncle and my grandmother used to read Ruth Montgomery and *Seth Speaks** when I was really little so I always had kind of a connection to that.

Connie's grandmother died when she was about 20. Since then, "sometimes when I do things I get a feeling that she's saying yes or no." Her uncle passed on 15 years ago. After that she started sensing communications from both of them.

> I get advice sometimes and I feel very grateful because the advice is really very good advice. When I was working, sometimes the administrators would ask you for information which you knew you didn't know, and I would say something like right off the cuff and it would be like my relatives were telling me. Then I would have to run and check it and make sure I was accurate. And there was no reason in the world why I should have that piece of information. It was like I'd hear someone feeding me this. I don't recall any time when I've taken the information and used it that it's been wrong.
>
> I don't have any sense that I'm holding them here, for whatever reason they maintain contact. My uncle and my grandmother were very protective of me. I think I had more contact with my uncle when I was working and used to have to work with technical information. He was incredibly intelligent so I think that he probably was there to help me, probably every couple of months or so.
>
> It's funny, they always used to call me Constance. Every once in a while I'll just hear, "Constance." I think, "What?" I know that it's one of the two of them. Nowadays I'll be sitting on my deck in a state

---

* Ruth Montgomery wrote extensively on the occult. *Seth Speaks* is one of several books said to have been channeled by Jane Roberts from an entity originally born in Atlantis who subsequently had a series of human lives.

of meditation and I get these little messages like, We're here, You're fine, Don't worry.

Like Connie, Jerry had a highly stressful childhood but was very much a survivor. (Recent findings, which I discuss in Chapter 16, suggest that trauma early in life often serves to create sensitives, people who are particularly able to receive messages that come via paranormal routes.) When Jerry was 17, he served with distinction as a Marine on Iwo Jima. For a time during the Vietnam War he was a journalist for *Life*. He broke with that magazine over what he viewed as its less than conscientious reporting of that conflict, then went on to have a successful career as an educator. Now in his seventies, he is a good-hearted bulldog of a man who campaigns to improve conditions for the needy in his county.

Jerry married the love of his life, Jenny, after each of them had had two children by a previous marriage. They had one more child together. Then, tragically, Jenny died and Jerry was left to raise five children without her. A couple of months after her death, Jerry started sensing Jenny's presence at night after the kids were asleep.

> I'd get in bed and she'd come and we'd talk about the kids. Startled me the first night, you know. Startled me that first night. Never saw her, just a telepathic thing. She'd give me advice about the kids, what to do. She seemed to know what we were doing and how we were living and so forth. She'd give me advice about Marie, about something I didn't know about her. And Josie, and Doug and Mike and so forth. And this went on, believe it or not, till the first four kids were majority age. When they were old enough and left home. I haven't heard from her since.

By the time the first four children were grown, Jerry had once again remarried. He and his third wife raised his youngest daughter together. Still his memories of Jenny remained vivid to him.

> You know the thing that I think about as I get older, Jenny knew what was going on with the kids that I didn't know. For instance, she told me that Josie would steal things. She'd steal from kids in school and from me. It was just her insecurities, is all. So I'd go to Josie and

she would deny it. Now Josie tells me it was all true. Jenny told me lots of things. You know, Marie had had a fight or Doug was unhappy and wanted to go back to his mother. Things like that. And she'd tell me, "I'm waiting for you, I'll be waiting for you." Of all the things when I die, gee, I want to see Jenny again.

Sylvia, 38, is tall, slim and leggy with blue eyes, striking cheekbones and light brown hair. She is a reiki practitioner and a singer-songwriter. When she was two, she was taken from a loving foster mother and adopted by a prosperous family in the New York area. Sylvia has no memories of her natural mother from that time. But as she grew older, she realized from vivid dreams that her natural mother "was no longer on this earth." Since she's eager to locate relatives and learn more about her birth family, she has asked me to supply her full birth name, Sylvia Alda, here. If anyone recalls anything that might be of interest to Sylvia, please contact me through my publisher or my website and I'll do my best to relay the information to her. Here is her story.

The first dream that I really remember, I was probably around 19 years of age. I had already had my first child and my cat had had kittens. I was gonna give them away to everyone and my birth mother came to me in a dream.

She's very serious and shorter than me, and her hair done under in a long pageboy going to the neck. In the dream she came and sat in the backseat of a car with me while someone else was driving and she told me, "Those kittens are all sick, they're all gonna die." And I didn't believe her, I was horrified. My reaction was so strong that the dream ended. Then when I woke up I was like, I wish I could have accepted that because I know that was my mother. I knew beyond a shadow of a doubt that that was my mother. And sure enough, those cats died. They had something that was incurable already.

The next time she came to me, I'd already had my three kids and I didn't feel right in my solar plexus area but I didn't want to go to the doctor. I don't like doctors at all, I've always taken care of myself. But I had a dream where she lay down right beside me and this plug of mucus came out of me and she was looking at it and she was saying, "You've got to get this checked out because it's not right." And again I didn't want to believe her and I was horrified and I woke up. But I did make a doctor's appointment and I went and checked on it and I actually had to have surgery for a growth. It's a good thing I caught it.

When my biological mother comes to me, it's always something I don't want to hear. It's helpful but it's not comforting.

Not all informational experiences relate to such somber matters. Alice, 55, has worked in museums as an educator and administrator and now works for an exhibit design company. When she was around 30, she had a joyous experience which enriched her sense of her family's roots. A Westerner, she was visiting Middletown, NY for the first time.

I was excited about going to Middletown. I'd never been there and my grandmother was from there. We parked near a bookstore we were planning to visit. I got out of the car and I just *felt* my grandmother was there and it was completely unexpected. She had been dead for about 4 years. So I said to my husband, "Well, you go on in and I'll join you shortly."

I just stood there and it was as if she were talking to me. I didn't really hear her words but the message that I got was, "This is where I grew up and my house is around the corner and up the street." So I went around the corner and up the street and it was this old street with like a railing. It went up a hill and there were all these old houses, probably from the turn of the century at least. There was a steep dropoff down the slope of the hill so there was a railing along the sidewalk, very distinctive.

I stopped in front of one house and it was like she was saying to me, "Well, this is my house." I just took it all in, it was fabulous. I really felt connected to her. It was really cool—and completely unexpected. So when I got home from my trip, I called my mother and I told her what had happened and she said, "Yah, that was the house." It was no surprise—I expected it to be the house. I mean, I didn't go there with my mother and say, "Is it this house?" But when I described the whole thing to her, she said, "Yah, that was the house."

Sometimes contacts with spirits have a farcical side. Anna, whose death coincidence was quoted in the previous chapter, had this experience a couple of days after her Aunt Katie died. She and her husband, along with several cousins, were staying at Katie's home for a few days.

> I look like her, so people always thought I was her daughter and we have so many personality traits that are identical. Among other things, she was a chocoholic and so am I. So anyhow, somewhere in the middle of the night I woke up and I had this huge urge for chocolate and I tried to tell myself, go back to sleep because you get fat if you eat in the middle of the night, you know. And I couldn't.
>
> I went downstairs and I went to the kitchen and as I tried to turn the lights on, instead of the lights coming on, they were blinking. They were like flickering and I had the thought of Oh my gosh, that's like Morse code but I don't know how to read it. And so inside of my head I thought, Is that you, Katie? And if so, where's the chocolate? And all of a sudden my eyes, or my attention was drawn to my right, and sort of beside or behind me where the pantry was. I opened the doors and I didn't see it, but all of a sudden I knew to look on the second shelf on the bottom in the back. Katie happened to be a diabetic and she was not supposed to have chocolate but that was where her stash was. I felt so tickled, I felt like she was there.
>
> The next night I woke up again in the middle of the night. I had the thought of wanting chocolate but I made up my mind I wasn't going to have it. But I did go downstairs and the lights did the same thing, they flickered. I did not have any sense of communication the second night like I did the first. It just was the lights. I told my husband about it and the next morning he tried the lights. He did all sorts of stuff. And they worked just fine. It had nothing to do with the electricity.

The next two accounts deal with one complicated event that resembles Anna's story in a couple of ways but starts off from a much darker place. After John was murdered when he was 19, his mother, his sister Sara and his half-sister, Spring, shared in a multi-faceted experience that proved to them that his spirit had survived and was reaching out to them. Early in my research study, I interviewed Spring, 26, a teacher. Here's the story she told me.

> I was visiting Angela, his mom, and Sara was there. She was watching videos in the other room and we were talking in the kitchen. She came into the kitchen and said, "Have you seen my

Rocky Horror Picture Show video?" And we said, "No, we don't know where it is." And so she went upstairs and Angela and I kept talking and suddenly the light in the kitchen got brighter and Angela said, "That's strange, that's never happened before." And she went and checked the knobs. You know, we turned them and all and she said, "It's all the way up, it's very strange. But it's no big deal." And then Sara came back down, all out of breath, and she said, "Oh my gosh," and of course we thought she was gonna talk about these lights that got brighter and she said, "You'll never believe what happened. I was upstairs and I was looking for my video and I just stopped and I said, 'John, show me where the video is,' and I reached my hand in the closet and I pulled it right out."

It was her room then, but it used to be his room. We were just so surprised because she came down immediately after the lights happened and this other thing happened for her, so our sense was, there was John doing that.

A few months later, I got a chance to interview Sara, Spring's 19 year-old half-sister, a college student and professional musician who lives in another state. She gave me a slightly different version of Spring's story.

I was looking for a video in my room. It wasn't Rocky Horror. My sister was wrong about that. It was a little cartoon that my brother had given me a long time ago. Anyway, I'd been looking for it for a really long time. And I was kind of frantic because it was really important to me. Johnny had given it to me. And I was searching every piece of my room, and finally I was like, "Johnny, just help me find it, please. Help me. Tell me where it is." And then I got this idea that it was in my closet. And I opened it up and opened up this weird box in the very bottom, and went to the bottom of the box on the left-hand side and pulled out the video. It was just like sitting there. Because I had no clue it was there at all. I hadn't seen it in a long time. So I really thought that he had like tuned into me at that point.

I guess while that happened, my mom and my sister were downstairs, and they said the lights got brighter. And I guess her lights don't really get brighter. She had them on all the way. So I ran downstairs. I was like, "Oh, I just found the video," and they were like, "Wow, the lights just got brighter."

Charlie is the college professor quoted in the previous chapter. After his mother died, he often sensed that she was communicating with him—but skeptic that he was, he looked for *proof* that what he sensed was founded in reality. One day when he was out running for exercise, twin incidents which he experienced within a matter of seconds convinced him that he wasn't just imagining things.

> One time when I was out running, in my left ear I heard Mom say, "Watch out." And just a couple seconds later, a little girl on a tricycle did a U-turn right into me. Now, it wasn't really dangerous, like I would get hurt, or like the little girl would get hurt either. But it was just very odd that she took this little U-turn toward me. I'd never seen anybody do that in the whole maybe year I was living in that neighborhood. But I get synchronicities in twos. I seem to be so skeptical that I need two hits on the head with a little hammer. "Wake up, Charlie, something's really happening."
>
> So about 10 seconds later, I turn the corner. Maybe not even 10 seconds, but it was definitely in a different spot because I turned the corner and nobody could see from one spot to the other. And after I turned the corner, I heard "Watch out" again. And this time, a boy riding a bicycle—the first was a little girl on a tricycle—this boy did the exact same maneuver of a U-turn right into me. And again, not really in a dangerous way, but it was obvious to me that there was a connection between the "watch out" and the maneuver.
>
> I didn't think that I was really being warned. It's just like it was a demonstration, not a serious warning. And the fact that it happened twice in a row like that was, to me, so much of a confirmation that I couldn't believe it was just a coincidence. They were such parallel events, those warnings and those two U-turns. And like I say, I get things in twos all the time.

Laura, 42, is a mortgage broker. Less than a year before I interviewed her, her husband, Dave, committed suicide after a long battle with depression. For a time, trying to relive the joyous highs of his youth, he'd started taking hallucinogens like some he'd given up completely 20 years before. But these forays into drug use only heightened his sense of unworthiness in the sight of God.

Before he died he told their mutual friend, Steve, "If anything ever happens to me, take care of Laura." After Dave's death, her relationship with Steve deepened—though she still continued to grieve for her husband. She and their daughter, Janie, often sensed that he was in touch with them.

On Dave's birthday seven months later, Laura and her 22 year-old daughter, Janie, had *interlocking* contact experiences with him that helped heal their pain and helped other family members as well. At this time, Laura was in Oregon while Janie was in Hawaii visiting her father's mother and sisters.

It was a day that was just topsy-turvy. Janie and I were going to talk on the phone but my own emotions hit me so much harder than I had expected on his birthday, that when I left work I elected not to go home. I had dinner out by myself. I just needed to be alone. It was a feeling of I just have to take care of me as the wife, I don't have any energy left to give as the mother. And after a while I felt a sense of peace at that.

No sooner had I gotten that sense of centering, I was driving along by the lake, when I felt this touch on my cheek. My husband used to take the side of his hand and stroke my cheek with his fingers. And then all along my right arm, driving, it was like electricity was making the hair stand out on my arm. And it was weird to me because I didn't have that feeling on my other arm, just the side that I perceived was near Dave. I knew immediately it was Dave 'cause I have sensed him several times. This time was so vividly clear. It was like there was a mist that was all around and then it drew in and became more concentrated until it was focused right next to me. Like if you filmed dry ice and it was all going out, you could run the film backwards.

I was thrilled that he was there and comforted—but it was his birthday and I was all distraught about this. Still I had this feeling that he was affirming me. Like, yeah, you're doing the right thing, don't worry about Janie. I wept because I was so thankful to feel him there. I thanked him. Then I asked him, "Could you do me a favor? Could you go out and see Janie today? It would mean a lot to her."

I'm out driving by the lake making this request to him as if it's okay. My religious thoughts on this are really turned upside down. *[For many years, Laura and Dave were missionaries for a fundamentalist church that believed suicides faced eternal damnation.]* And then I was getting ready to turn down the road to Steve's. And I kind of looked over to where I felt he was and I said, "You can come with me if you want." And I'm going, this is weird. But it was as clear as a bell. He said, "No, you need to go on with your life, I gotta go see Janie."

I got down to Steve's and there were a couple of other friends there and I told them what had happened, and they're of course looking at me like I've got two heads. And I said, I guarantee you that when I get home there's going to be a message from my daughter saying that daddy had appeared, that he'd shown up. And sure enough, I got home that night about twelve or twelve-thirty, and there was a message. Not a lot of detail on it, just, "Mom, I had a weird experience. Call me."

So I call her up and she was kind of withdrawn initially. His family had been asking for more details as to what had led up to him choosing to commit suicide and she was between a rock and a hard place because some of those issues are not really dinner table conversation. So she was voicing this out, trying to get what my take was on it. The bottom line was I said, "You have to do what you feel is right no matter what anybody else on the planet thinks. This is the one message since daddy died that is holding me to the ground like I've never had before. Trust your own intuition to do what's right and you will have peace regardless of what anybody else says or does." And she goes, "Oh, mama, that's almost exactly word for word what daddy told me."

And I started to cry and I said, "Tell me what happened." She goes, "I went down to the beach. I took some of his ashes like we said and I was sitting on the beach feeling all forlorn. I was disappointed because he hadn't shown up yet and it was his birthday and here it was sunset." Dave said he would send us love letters in the sunsets. She says, "I figured, well, daddy must just be with mamma, it was always kind of their day. I felt like a second class citizen." And she was grappling with this question about whether she should reveal more of what Dave's situation was to his relatives.

All of a sudden, she felt him kind of sit beside her. She goes, "It felt like he was holding me and reassuring me. And that's what he said to me, just follow your heart. Just stay centered to that and stay true to that and tell 'em whatever you feel is right." A few days later she called me back and told me what had happened from that. It was wonderful.

She went ahead and told the family and that really helped them to go, "Oh, okay." And also to be able to tell her, "Oh heck, Dave's not alone. This other family member had the same sort of situation happen with them." And for Janie it was, "Oh good, Daddy wasn't so weird after all."

That sunset happened in Hawaii between six-thirty and quarter to seven. That was nine-thirty to quarter to ten here. Which was when I had driven down to Steve's and told him about what happened, it was exactly the same time. So it was like, Dave got in my car and then he went over to Hawaii.

Laura's contact experiences have had a transforming effect on her religious beliefs. In the next chapter we look at the wealth of faith traditions that acknowledge the reality of contact with spirits.

4

How World Religions View Survival of the Spirit

LET'S SUPPOSE THAT AFTER-DEATH CONTACTS are nothing new. Let's suppose that ever since our forebears countless millennia ago started dressing themselves in animal skins or platted grasses, since they started shaping stone tools and taming fire, studying the stars and scraping images of their world on the walls of caves and cliffs, they sensed contacts with their dead—contacts not much different from those described in this book. Let's suppose too that sometimes other strange and wonderful adventures came to members of their wandering bands, personal events that blessed them with a sense of something beyond the material: near-death experiences, out-of-body experiences, or mystical visions. What would the stories they shared with their companions have led these primal peoples to believe?

Wouldn't they have felt instructed that some part of the self can survive after death? How better can we account for the eighty thousand year-old graves of Neanderthal humans whose bodies were buried with food and tools and laid out with attention to the east-west path of the sun, which each night dies into darkness and each morning is reborn? Symbolism was not invented in our own era. It seems to spring from some enduring human essence.

In a cross-cultural study of grief and mourning, Prof. Paul Rosenblatt of the University of Minnesota evaluated the "ghost beliefs" of 66 societies including our own. Only one, the Masai—

about which only limited data were available—was judged to have no belief in spirits as manifestations of specific dead persons. Our own differed from most of the others by viewing "ghosts as a topic for jokes, fanciful films, and fiction. To admit that one has perceived a ghost or the action of a ghost is to invite being labeled as ignorant, superstitious, irrational, or hallucinating. It is sobering," Rosenblatt and his colleagues observed, "to find American culture so much in the minority on this issue." Societies from all over the world—Apaches and Caribs in the Western hemisphere, Hokkien speakers in Taiwan, the Azande of the Sudan, and a farflung sampling of Polynesians—shared belief in spirits.

Such beliefs often involve critical thinking. For instance, describing the beliefs of the Trobriand Islanders who lived off the coast of New Guinea, the noted anthropologist Bronislaw Malinowski reported that they made a distinction not unlike that made by many of my informants regarding contacts perceived in dreams. "Not all dreams about the departed are regarded as true.... Real spirits always come with a purpose and under conditions in which they can properly be expected. Thus, if a recently dead person appears in sleep to a surviving relative, giving him some important message or announcing his death at a distance—such a dream is true." Clearly these people had experienced death coincidences—announcements of death at a distance—and viewed them as a common form of contact with the dead.

When we look at after-death contacts—and near-death experiences and mystical visions—we are looking at the stuff from which religions are born. For what, after all, are religions but systematic explanations that people create for the world they perceive around them?

To say this is not to deny the divine source that many of these explanations may have. Quite the contrary. History abounds in stories of people reputed to be seers or saints or avatars. Personally, since some of my own experiences have led me to believe totally in the reality of divine powers, I'm inclined to credit many of those stories. Recently a Tibetan monk told me that, according to his tradition, every hundredth boy is born to be a wise man, every hundredth girl is born to be an angel. Who can say for certain?

Maybe he's right. Nonetheless, as we look at the variety of the world's religions, we are reminded of the cautionary wisdom of First Corinthians 13:

> As for prophecies, they will pass away; as for tongues, they will cease; as for knowledge, it will pass away. For our knowledge is imperfect and our prophecy is imperfect; but when the perfect comes, the imperfect will pass away. When I was a child, I spoke like a child, I reasoned like a child; when I became a man, I gave up childish ways. For now we see as in a mirror dimly, but then face to face. Now I know in part; then I shall understand fully. . . .

Only after death, the apostle Paul tells us, can people know fully and perfectly. Little wonder that over the millennia, different peoples have come up with varying explanations of what follows after each of us mortals closes our eyes on earth for the final time. Nonetheless, certain themes recur again and again, not only among so-called "primitive" cultures but among some of the great religions of the world. Reincarnation and ancestor worship stand out among these themes—and central to both of them is belief in survival after death of some part of the human spirit.

When after my husband died, his Hindu friend, an engineer, told me that it was normal for a dead person's spirit to wander the earth freely for a time, I wasn't all that surprised. I was aware, as most Americans are, that Hindus—however well-educated and competent in dealing with this material world—believe in reincarnation. This presupposes that some essential part of each personality travels beyond death through an intermediate stage, then enters a new body—not necessarily human—to be born again.

Buddhists too, I knew, believed in reincarnation and I'd heard that in some fashion the Chinese practiced ancestor worship. I'd even heard that contemporary Chinese particularly resented their government's limitations on family size because, according to their traditions, only *sons* can properly perform some of the duties due to ancestors. If an observant Chinese family's first child is a daughter, they feel obliged to keep having children until they have at least one son. What I didn't know back in the eighties when my husband died was how widely religious practices that stem from belief in spirit survival have arisen independently around the world. They were even commonplace in Europe before the Christian era.

Caesar in his *Gallic Wars* attributed the fearlessness of Celtic warriors to their belief that after death their souls would pass into another body. The Gauls customarily threw letters addressed to their dead onto funeral pyres. Archeologists have found in the funeral practices of the ancient Celts, Germans and Scandinavians evidence that they believed in the immortality of the spirit and in a continuing relationship between the dead and the living. As *The Encyclopedia of Religion* points out: "Evidence is abundant, including ... burials in coffins marked with solar symbols.... Everything in these graves speaks in the symbolic language of the afterlife: the preservation of skulls, the location of graves near the living, bodies turned to face the house, and the inclusion of the dead person's possessions."

Among some of the Slavs of Eastern Europe and Russia, belief in supernatural beings—both good and evil—has survived into modern times. This part of the world has, after all, sired popular stories of werewolves and vampires as well as more agreeable nature spirits. Writing in the 1950s a Slavic scholar described *domoviks*, domestic guardians which were thought to inhabit each home. Peasant practices, he said, "suggest that the being who is worshipped as a household god is really the spirit of the ancestor, or founder of the family, who ... still attends to the interests of his descendants.... At the festivals held in commemoration of ancestors, honors are paid to the household spirit as well." In Scandinavia, he reported, some people still offered small gifts of food to their home's protective spirits, thought to be the souls of dead ancestors.

In 1999, National Public Radio (NPR) aired a report on the revival of traditional beliefs in Siberia. Syanna Num Soiava, a professional woman coming home to visit her parents, was interviewed about her plan to visit a shaman. (Shamans are the specially trained and respected clairvoyant/healers found in tiny communal societies all over the world. The word "shaman" itself comes from a Mongol language spoken in Eastern Siberia.) Before Syanna's return, she explained, the local shaman had carried out a ceremony on an ancestor's grave for the family. "The shaman lady was talking with spirits about all living relatives and their children. My mother asked about me, and this great ancestral spirit told that I need to make a purification ceremony." NPR went on to provide a few sound bytes from that six hour-long ceremony in which the shaman, in keeping with Buddhist practice, rang a bell to call the spirits and then made offerings to them of tea, milk and vodka.

The Mari, an indigenous Finnish people who have maintained their traditional practices into the present era, believe that after death the spirit remains near the corpse. A feast is given in its honor during the memorial service, then the spirit is ceremonially led to the grave. These Finns, though ostensibly converted to Christianity, give the corpse gifts for other dead members of the family and "believe that the living and the dead form a family that is cemented together at the funeral and the memorial services.... [Their language] carries traces of ideas about an underground abode of the dead and the dead person's continuing his work."

There is more than a little resemblance between Mari beliefs and those that characterize most African traditional religions— religions that must have arisen independently many thousands of miles away. For instance, Africans may entrust to the newly deceased messages for those already on the other side, and they view the spirits of their dead as continuing parts of their community.

Across the sub-Saharan region of the continent, adherents of traditional African religions practice ancestor worship—though not all their dead are honored equally. Such status is more often granted to community leaders—chiefs, priests and such—or to those who have lived a good life and reached a ripe old age. Africans also tend to agree that there is one Supreme Being, but they envision him—God's masculinity is not to be questioned!— as being so lofty and proud that no individual dare pray to him directly. The Kikuyu believe that a family group praying together and led by the family's senior person, typically the father or grandfather, may appeal to their chief deity, Ngai, for help. Other tribes pray for the spirits of their ancestors, or lesser deities, to intercede with their supreme deity for them. Thus in an obser-

vant Zulu village, each hut and particularly the hut of the head-
man boasts a special place for communing with ancestral spirits,
and part of the enclosure within the village's circle of huts is used
for ceremonies directed to the ancestors. Similarly, each Yoruba
home has a family shrine where the head of the family performs
rites to seek their help and approval.

Educated Africans, ostensibly converted to Christianity or
Islam and far removed from their ancestral villages, often cling to
such traditional observances. What's more, the ancient religious
heritage of the Yoruba lives on not only in its homeland, Nigeria,
but in Cuba, Brazil and even in parts of the United States. Yoruban
slaves forced to convert to Catholicism in Latin America used
Catholic saints as proxies for their own deities and blended the two
religions into what in now called Santería. It is still widely practiced
by Hispanics, most of them not of African descent.

In the ancient world of the Middle East, to which much of
Western culture traces its roots, a long sequence of peoples built
their rituals and their faiths around belief in the spirit's survival
after death. The pyramids and the Pyramid Texts testify to the early
Egyptian belief that, after death, the pharaoh would fly to the
heavens where he would reign as a star or as a companion of the sun
god. By the second millennium before Christ, more democratic
beliefs had taken hold. It was thought that if after death a com-
moner was mummified, his or her soul could come and go at will
from its preserved body and might leave its tomb during the day
and move among the living here on earth, returning to rest in its
tomb at night. Since the Egyptians found much of joy in everyday
life, they believed that many a soul would choose to visit often
among the living. The Mesopotamians, who lived in what is now
Iraq, had a darker view of the world. They viewed the underworld
rather than the sky as the site of the afterlife and scrupulously
honored their dead out of fear that disgruntled ghosts might injure
the living.

A friend of mine whose parents came from Greece once
laughingly told me, "If you have five Greeks in a room, you have six
opinions." Apparently in the ancient Hellenic world, similar inde-
pendence of mind was the rule. According to Homer, only aristo-

crats made it into the Grecian paradise, Elysium. Later, while many believed that death led to perpetual, dreary exile beyond the river Styx in the underworld, some great philosophers—Pythagoras and Plato, in particular—believed that immortal souls might undergo purification in Hades and then be reborn into new human bodies again and again. On a less abstract level, each year at a popular festival, Greeks put out pots of cooked fruit for the dead of the family. The inscription on an ancient grave marker found on the island of Rhodes documents belief there in survival of the spirit and in the possibility of enduring contact with a beloved lost spouse:

> If there is a highest praise in the world befitting a woman, with this died Kalliarista, daughter of Phileratos, for wisdom and virtue. For this reason her husband Damocles set up this stele as a memorial of love, *and may a benevolent spirit follow him for the rest of his life.* [Italics added.]

The rulers of the ancient Roman world, like those of our own day, were more interested in the crafts of law, engineering and war than in philosophy and questions of the soul. Skeptical and materialistic, their interest in enduring verities expressed itself more in building aqueducts, roads and coliseums than in metaphysical inquiry. Eclecticism may have been their saving grace. Even as, during the last two centuries of the pre-Christian era, they extended their empire over the great Greek cities, they borrowed much Greek culture. In matters religious, the Romans hedged their bets.

From the 13th to the 21st of February, they celebrated an annual feast of the dead which they called "Parentalia." According to the poet Ovid, small offerings left on the path to a tomb would suffice: a few violets, a tile wreathed in flowers, bread soaked in wine, or a sprinkling of salt or grain. On February 22nd, the family gathered together and the spirits of their departed relatives were believed to visit them. During contrasting rituals observed by the Romans in May, evil spirits were thought to be expelled.

How did our own Judeo-Christian beliefs regarding spirit survival evolve? According to most of the Old Testament, She'ol, a dreary world of shadows much like Hades, was thought to be the final destination of the dead. Nonetheless in pre-Biblical times the ancient Israelites had put food, weapons and other provisions in graves. Apparently the custom of symbolically feeding the dead survived into the time of Moses. In Deuteronomy 26:12, such behavior is mentioned in a backhanded way: "When you have finished paying all the tithe of your produce . . . then you shall say before the Lord your God . . . 'I have not eaten of the tithe . . . or *offered any of it to the dead.*'" [Italics added.]

Furthermore, though King Saul is said to have exiled mediums from Israel, the Bible (I Samuel 28) tells us that, when threatened by a great army of Philistines, he disguised himself and sought out a medium still secretly practicing her art in the area. This poor lady whom the Bible never dignifies with a name, is referred to in the King James version as the "witch of Endor."

At Saul's bidding, she conjures up for him the spirit of his dead mentor, Samuel. Then, psychic that she is, she senses the king's real identity and cries out, "Why have you deceived me?" Saul, hardly in a mood to exile her just then, responds, "Have no fear. What do you see?" The woman from Endor sees "a god coming out of the earth," an old man wrapped in a robe.

With dire accuracy, Samuel tells King Saul that soon he will be killed in battle. "Tomorrow you and your sons will be with me." Saul falls to the ground, not only because he's terrified by what he's just heard but because he hasn't eaten for the past twenty-four hours. When the medium learns from Saul's servants how famished he is, like a good Jewish mother she slaughters a fatted calf of her own, whips up some unleavened bread, and sets a hospitable table for Saul and his servants. In this, as in her mediumship, she does a good and generous job.

Before the Arabs, ancient kinsmen of the Hebrews, were converted to Islam, they too clearly believed in spirit survival. They supplied their dead with food and drink. If they came upon an acquaintance's grave, they greeted the person by name and thought it not unlikely that they would receive an answer. According to Islamic scholar, M. S. Seale, owls that fluttered by were thought to contain the spirits of the departed. A poetess, Layla, visiting the grave of her poet-lover, "dared question the belief that the deceased returned one's salutation, despite the fact that her lover had himself said so in one of his poems. At this bold denial, an owl appeared and flew straight into her face. Layla dropped dead." Echoes of this extraordinary story abound in Chapter 11 of this book. Several of the people I interviewed had experienced symbolic actions by birds that they took to be after-death communications. Fortunately all of them survived to tell the tale.

In the closing centuries of the pre-Christian era, Jewish thought about the afterlife underwent a transformation. In 322 B.C., Alexander the Great conquered Palestine. Alexander had been tutored by Aristotle and came from Macedonia which bordered Greece on the northwest. For almost two hundred years thereafter, the region was governed by Hellenized rulers—first Macedonians, then Syrians. Palestine's Jews were so strongly influenced by this environment that many of them forgot their own language. That's why, during the third century B.C., the Hebrew Bible was translated into Greek. (This is the Septuagint translation which, according to tradition, was completed by 70 Hebrew scholars in as many days.) Soon Jewish religious thinkers were influenced by other belief systems in the intellectual ferment of the Middle East. None had a greater impact on them than Zoroastrianism.

Now Zoroastrianism is hardly a popular buzzword. Alas, its name is too long and it's forever doomed to bring up the rear in alphabetical order. Nonetheless I'm going to say quite a bit about it because much of what we associate with Western religion stems from this obscure faith which originated in Iran and which in 1976 was estimated to have just 130,000 adherents. As of that date, Zoroastrianism was still being practiced by a poor minority in Iran and by disproportionately influential Parsee communities in India and Pakistan. (Their name, Parsee, means Persian.)

Late in the second millennium before the Christian era, Zoroaster reformed the worship of many gods—akin to ancient Hinduism—then accepted in Iran. A priest and a prophet, he preached that there was just one supreme deity. Several immortals who formerly had been worshipped as gods in their own right were instead merely archangels serving Ahura Mazda, the one Wise Lord, who lived in a realm of light. (Early in the twentieth century, some learned industrialist recruited "Mazda" as a brand name for light bulbs.)

Another name for Zoroaster is Zarathushtra. If that sounds familiar but slightly wrong, you may recall that the German philosopher Nietzsche wrote a book called *Thus Spake Zarathustra;* Richard Strauss composed a tone poem of the same name; then Stanley Kubrick used this same tone poem as background music for his film, *2001, A Space Odyssey.* Scholars on ancient Iran sometimes get huffy about Nietzsche's spelling of Zarathushtra's name so let's sidestep that problem and call him Zoroaster.

Central to the faith that Zoroaster taught is a cosmic battle between the forces of good and evil. Though this concept figures largely in the New Testament, it is virtually absent from the Old. According to Zoroaster, Ahura Mazda has a wicked adversary, Angra Mainyu. Just as Satan is defined by Christians as a son of God who has rebelled against him, Angra Mainyu is one of the twin sons of the Wise Lord. However unlike the omnipotent God of the Judeo-Christian tradition, Ahura Mazda needs human help to defeat his wayward son. Those who in life strive for the right win immediate reward after death in heaven.

In contrast to earlier Indo-Iranian beliefs that only high ranking men—preferably princes, warriors or priests—could hope to attain paradise, Zoroaster taught that even women and servants could be among the blessed. When a person dies, his or her soul lingers near the body for three nights. (This belief—like many others around the world—seems to stem from the wealth of contact experiences sensed soon after the death of a loved one.) After this short stay, according to Zoroaster, the soul is carried away to judgment at the Chinvat Bridge between earth and heaven. Righteous souls are swept along by a fragrant wind and a beautiful girl and ecstatically cross the bridge to paradise. Souls that in life acted wickedly are confronted by a hag and buffeted by stench. That fateful bridge shrinks under their feet to the width of a razor's edge and bad guys topple off the bridge into the world of the damned. As for those ambivalent folk whose thoughts, words and deeds haven't been predominantly either good or bad, they wind up in a kind of limbo, a shadow place much like She'ol or Hades where there is neither joy nor torment.

Shortly before the time of Christ, pivotal Jewish thinkers started putting forward visions of the afterlife that echoed those of this Iranian faith. Until then Jews believed that Heaven was reserved for just two holy immortals, Enoch and Elijah, and there was no Hell beyond the shadow world of She'ol. Now the anonymous authors of the First Book of Enoch—long studied by theologians but never included in the Bible—affirmed that the spirits of the upright and elect, once freed from their bodies, would dwell in joy in a "garden of righteousness." (The word "paradise"—*pardes* in Hebrew—stems from an ancient Iranian term for an enclosed park or orchard.) Similarly 1 Enoch introduced to Jewish thought, the concept of eternal damnation in Gehenna, an "abyss ... full of fire."

Many other precepts of the Zoroastrians sound curiously familiar to anyone brought up on Judeo-Christian traditions. From the earliest days of their faith over 3,000 years ago, they believed that at some climactic time the world would face a Last Judgment when the earth would "give up the bones of the dead." Rivers of fire would flow like lava and all humanity would have to pass through them. This culminating ordeal would wipe the wicked from the earth while the blessed would regain their resurrected bodies and live on forever in perfect bliss in a purified world.

When Zoroaster was preaching his message, he seems to have believed that the end of the world was close at hand but he didn't think that he himself would live to see it. He therefore prophesied that another great leader, the Saoshyant, would come after him to lead humanity. Zoroaster's followers came to trust that the Saoshyant would be born of a virgin. At the fated time, she would be impregnated with the prophet's own seed, miraculously preserved in a lake where she bathed.

One last intriguing point about this little discussed tradition. Most of the priestly class of those early Zoroastrians came from a tribe called the Magi. Throughout the Hellenistic world, this term was used for Eastern astrologers and interpreters of dreams or, more generally, for men of wisdom who could fathom things divine.

To this day, Zoroastrians believe that the families of the newly dead play an important role in their progress. Using the sacred fires that are central to Zoroastrian worship, they make ritual offerings frequently during the first year after a loved one's death so that the traveling soul is properly fed and clothed. Then, in an annual observance on the last night of each year, the faithful celebrate the Feast of All Souls. Spirits are thought to return to their earthly homes at sunset and leave again as the sun rises on New Year's Day.

A special class of spirits, the fravashis, are helpers and protectors. Apparently first thought of as departed heroes, fravashis came to be thought of as something like Valkyries, female winged beings who could help bring rain, could assure that families had children, and in time of battle, would fight beside their descendants. Viewed through Western eyes, belief in such spirit presences doesn't just document belief in survival after death. Fravashis also seem to foreshadow guardian angels.

Over the millennia, since the days of our Stone Age forebears, people have agreed that some part of the human essence can survive death. Cultures disagree about the details. Do all spirits or only a select few go on to become "ancestors" who systematically interact with the living? Do spirits face judgment immediately after death? If so, what alternatives may confront them thereafter? Are some souls simply expunged? Or are they reborn into different bodies? And if so, are they always *human* bodies? And if there is a Last Judgment, what form will this apocalypse take?

The cosmic theories go on and on. I won't argue here for any one in preference to another. But thinking people should recognize that *all these theories are intellectual artifacts just as real in their way as physical artifacts like stone tools, shards of pottery or ancient idols. They testify to almost unanimous belief from the dawn of time that something of the human spirit can live on after death. Probably because, century after century, ordinary folks have sensed contact with loved ones who have passed on.*

Accounts of a cataclysmic flood abound in the legends of peoples around the world. No one scoffs when scientists seek concrete evidence for such a flood or offer theories about how one could have happened. Similarly, stories and art from many traditions have been pieced together to date ancient celestial events like comets. Why then is it unorthodox in the Western world to think contact with the spirits of the dead may be real?

Compulsive disbelievers argue that people cherish faith in life after death simply because they dread total extinction or prefer to imagine "pie in the sky when you die." But at best this is a fragmentary picture of what people really believe about the afterlife. Many traditions around the world have envisioned a paradise to which only the heroes or nobility could aspire. More commonly they've pictured hellish places where guiltier spirits went either for purification or permanent torment. Many of the people I interviewed said that, before they had a particular after-death contact, they'd been worrying about a departed loved one. Clearly, they were fearful that his or her spirit might be suffering. In fact, one of the most common messages that people receive in an after-death contact is, "I'm okay. Stop worrying about me."

Nowadays many of the people who consider themselves religious are alienated from conventional religion. According to a CNN/USA *Today*/Gallup poll conducted in 1994, 69% of Americans believed religion was losing influence in American life. Writing in 1995, the Gallup Organization reported that although 96% of Americans said they believed in "God or a universal spirit" and 88% said that religion was important in their lives, only 58% claimed to attend a church or synagogue as often as once a month. By 1998, more Americans (64%) expressed quite a lot of confidence in the military than in organized religion (59%). Yet 82% said they felt a need to experience spiritual growth.

Psi events like ADCs often lead people to rethink their personal faiths. Near death and out of body experiences, mystical moments of transcendent grace, sensing the infinite through "other ways of knowing"—all these can transform a person's inner life, enriching them and teaching them timeless, immaculate truths. When I asked the people I interviewed about their beliefs, a remarkable number said they considered themselves "spiritual, not religious."

Much of America seems to be trending this way. Yet a persistent taboo keeps people from sharing the spiritual insights they've gained. In the next chapter, we'll take a look at our culture's resistance to acknowledging the reality of contact with the dead.

5

Facing up to a Cultural Taboo

IN OUR WESTERN CULTURE, a three-pronged taboo discourages discussion of after-death contacts.

By far the most common reason why people keep mum about the psychic events in their lives is that they don't want others to think they've wigged out, lost their marbles, gone round the bend. Now that more and more TV programs, books and movies are dealing with psi, it's easy to think that personal reticence must be fading away. Not so. The problem is the *way* the media deal with psi. It's rarely viewed as commercial unless it's wildly sensational and if it's wildly sensational it's probably far from true. Only the occasional book or cable program faithfully reports the subtle ways that people usually sense the paranormal. Until this changes, most of the public will continue to view accounts of spirit contacts as "a topic for jokes, fanciful films and fiction."

Few of my interviewees have come from localities which are especially conservative or out-of-touch with contemporary life. About two-thirds of them live in or around Eugene, Oregon, a West Coast university town that boasts a significant minority of now solid citizens who, as counter-culture hippies in the seventies, moved north from the San Francisco Bay Area. For many years the local free paper has devoted a sizable section to ads concerning what they call Intuitive Arts. In Eugene, astrologers, energy healers, and various schools of psychics thrive. Nonetheless, here are typical responses I received in 1998 and 1999 when I asked my informants if they had told others about their psi experiences.

> I told several of my brothers. One time I told a neighbor and then I decided I wasn't going to tell people. He looked wild eyed at me. No, I haven't told too many people.

> Very few. Only people that I felt would be receptive and not look at me like I'm crazy, not judge me or look at me strangely.

> You start talking about this and it gives people the creeps. Even my girlfriend who I'm quite close to gets really uncomfortable if I talk too much about it. [This from a middle-aged married woman.]

> I don't talk about it with friends 'cause they'd just think you were freaky.

> I don't tell a whole lot of people because sometimes they look at you and then look for the exit. As if you escaped from the local mental ward or something.

A British psychologist, a widower whom I interviewed long distance via e-mail, summed up much of the syndrome in a few pithy words:

> Discussion is made very difficult by the psychiatric, atheistic assumption that almost everything that happens after bereavement, other than "recovering and getting on with your life," must be a hallucination. The religious view that forbids consideration of the nature of the afterlife or communication with spirits is also influential.

As a psychologist, my correspondent was well aware that many mentally ill people see and hear things that aren't really there. Their false perceptions are symptoms of disease. But by the same token, he knew that most of the men and women who *paranormally* perceive things which others don't perceive are perfectly well.

This distinction is of more than passing concern. The perceiver's welfare may depend on the judgment others make about his or her sanity. Recently a young professor confided in me that, a few months earlier, his seven year-old daughter had been troubled by sensations that her deceased aunt—who in life had been a highly disturbed person—was coming to her from time to time, urging her to act suicidally so she could join her aunt on the other side. "My wife and I were afraid to take her to a regular counselor," he said. "We were afraid she'd end up on meds." Fortunately one of their relatives suggested that he and his wife consult a talented sensitive. All the little girl had to do, the sensitive told her, was to firmly tell her aunt's spirit to go away. The little girl complied and her aunt's spirit stopped bothering her.

For a dismal contrast, consider a tale told to me by Joe McMoneagle, one of 61 perceivers I interviewed in 1998. Joe is a psychic celebrity, one of the world's most gifted remote viewers. A Vietnam veteran and career army man, for eighteen years he was "viewer no. 001" in a research project initiated by the C.I.A. and supported by the Army Intelligence and Security Command.

Remote viewing is a little known and almost inconceivable ability. It's closely related to the skills of some psychics, often consulted by the police, who if given a chance to handle the possessions of a missing person, can tell what's become of him or her. If you give remote viewers a sealed envelope with a photograph inside it, they're likely to be able to sketch the picture in detail and tell you what's been happening to whatever it represents. Sometimes map coordinates, longitude and latitude, do just as well.

Not surprisingly, Joe's talents have included other forms of clairvoyance. While he was stationed at embattled outposts in Vietnam, he would sense mortar attacks before they happened and duck into a bunker. His fellow soldiers soon started taking for the bunkers whenever they saw Joe headed that way. He also had near death and out of body experiences before such phenomena were described in the media. Somehow, as a young man, he taught himself to live a double life, keeping his psychic adventures secret from his associates in the military—until the military discovered how useful his talents might be for spying. His twin sister, now dead, made different choices which didn't serve her as well.

> My sister was as sensitive as I was and the problem was, when *she* started having visions or seeing things, she went to a classic psychia-

trist who immediately started giving her chemicals and drugs. From that point on, it was downhill. I have a lot of personal anger over that. If she had been lucky enough to have gotten a Jungian counselor, she might've been okay but she went to a psychiatrist who immediately said, "You're delusional, here take these drugs," and any time she got carried away, she was like hospitalized and was slammed with classical aversion therapy. . . . The help she sought turned out to be very destructive for her.

Judith Orloff—who is both a psychiatrist and a psychic—confirms this judgment. Doctors, she reports, tend to equate psychic awareness with psychosis. In their *Diagnostic and Statistical Manual IV,* "the Bible of the American Psychiatric Association ... it is referred to only as a symptom of mental disorder, a biochemical instability that needs to be wiped out by powerful antipsychotic drugs like Thorazine. . . . Unfortunately the overall sentiment among most mainstream physicians is that the psychic is nonexistent, a sham, or a disease."

In reality there's evidence that people who display heightened awareness of the paranormal are sounder mentally than most of their fellows. Shamans—the rigorously trained clairvoyant healers often found in tiny, pre-industrial societies—are "commonly described as displaying remarkable energy and stamina, unusual levels of concentration, control of altered states of consciousness, high intelligence, leadership skills, and a grasp of complex data, myths, and rituals."

Similarly, when almost 1500 Americans were polled about any mystical experiences they might have had, two-fifths responded that on at least one occasion they had "had the feeling of being very close to a powerful spiritual force" that seemed to lift them out of themselves. When these sometime mystics were tested for psychological well-being, the relationship between frequent ecstatic experiences and mental health was exceedingly high—higher than the designer of the test had found for any other group.

People who sense paranormal communication, whatever its route, may be receiving messages directed only to them. Quite a few of them, myself included, occasionally gain paranormal insights from material events which are readily perceptible to anyone else present—for instance, as described in this book's opening chapter: a light flashing, a can of seasonings fallen from a shelf, a kitchen grater lying on a counter. In Chapters 9-12, dozens of perceivers report symbolic meanings they gleaned from a wide variety of material events. Oftentimes the knowledge that came to them through the conventional five senses was supplemented telepathically.

I can't claim any sort of communication with the ghost of Louis Pasteur, telepathic or otherwise. Nonetheless I suspect that the good doctor who, in the mid-nineteenth century, fathered the science of microbiology would look kindly on this inquiry. For years he battled a scientific establishment which took it for granted (erroneously) that the spontaneous generation of life forms was possible—that maggots or eels or mice could appear where no parent creatures had been before—yet which chose to disbelieve that microorganisms too small for them to see could have mighty powers to curdle milk, spoil wine or, most important, cause illness. It took over two decades before the germ theory of disease which he had proven by rigorous experiments was generally accepted. Sadly enough, some health professionals who should know better, still seem less than mindful of its implications. A recent New York Times article headlined "Doctors Are Reminded, Wash Up!" reported that "only 17% of physicians treating patients in an intensive care unit washed their hands appropriately."

This brings us to the second prong of the taboo against sensing after-death contacts. For years no group more consistently opposed notions of psi and spirit survival than members of the medical-scientific establishment. According to one Gallup report, they were only about a quarter as likely as the rest of the public to believe that there was an afterlife or reincarnation or that it was possible to sense contact with the dead. But curiously enough, they were almost as likely as the general public to believe that life comparable to our own exists elsewhere in the universe. This, although there's far less evidence for any such thing than there is for paranormal phenomena.

Recently there have been some startling breakthroughs in the thinking of medical doctors, at least with respect to the impact of spirituality on healing. According to a recent survey of 2700 physicians, "81% of the respondents agreed that 'better clinical outcomes can result directly from a patient's spirituality' ... and a majority (57%) agreed that their own spirituality could be important." They were probably responding to the flood of evidence, gleaned from double-blind studies over the past couple of decades, which demonstrate that prayer can help cure human illness and can mitigate the effects of ailments from heart disease to AIDS. It can even foster the growth of plants and other life forms.

A group called Spindrift, cited by Dr. Larry Dossey, have "systematically done studies showing the ability of what they call 'prayer practitioners' to influence the course of simple biological systems. They will pray, for instance, for one batch of germinating seeds and not for another, then measure the germination rate of these groups. . . . They come out with numerical data to measure their results, and nothing is subjectively evaluated. These studies have shown beyond any doubt that prayer is effective."

Unfortunately the old guard of the medical profession continues to offer material explanations for spiritual events. As Raymond Moody wrote in 1999, "scientific skeptics, in their dealing with people who have had unusual, allegedly paranormal experiences, content themselves with pointing out that the experience wasn't what the person having it thought it was at all, but just misfiring neurons, a chemical imbalance, fantasy, or whatever." Moody is the psychiatrist whose book *Life after Life* first introduced the concept of the near-death experience. A couple of years ago, he observed to me that MDs often insist that near-death experiences result from a lack of oxygen in the brain—though he knew of many classic near-death experiences which involved no such thing. Sure enough, in an A & E special, "Beyond Death," shown on TV in July 2000, two medical people independently attributed the sensations of all NDEs to a shortage of either blood or oxygen in the brain.

A century ago, scientists tried to study contact with the dead by subjecting mediums to investigation under controlled conditions. Some of these poor ladies (almost all of the sensitives investigated were women) put up with an astonishing array of intrusions and indignities. These sometimes involved full body searches and chains. Despite the awkward conditions under which these mediums had to perform, some of the results they managed to achieve were startlingly convincing. Nonetheless, unrelenting skepticism from the bulk of the scientific community confounded most of these research efforts.

The trouble is, as soon as you try to study after-death contacts induced by a *medium* you're dealing with what social scientists call an intervening variable. Doubts arise that some fiendishly clever ruse might be involved—even though the researchers may not be able to detect it. That's why this book deals primarily with *spontaneous* contacts, experiences that have come when least expected to ordinary people with no professional stake in proving their sensitivity to the occult. All of them anonymous, all of them unpaid.

Of course, that vaunted "scientific method" is interpreted quite differently from one discipline to another. Astronomers can't do lab experiments on stars. Meteorologists can't do double-blind experiments on the weather. And archeologists have to rely on intuition as much as on chemical analysis to guess at the significance of what they find in their digs. Sometimes data laboriously analyzed in orthodox fashion turns out to prove something quite different when new tools come to hand. One case in point: DNA testing has led biochemists and geneticists to drastically redraw the tree of life. What once was thought to have three major branches is now seen as having five. Fungi like mushrooms are now classified as closer to animals than plants.

Furthermore, though ideally it's great to know *why* a particular medical treatment works before you use it, smallpox might have remained a worldwide scourge far longer than it did if back in the late 18th century an English surgeon named Edward Jenner hadn't noticed that milkmaids who got nodules on their hands from milking cows with a mild disease called cowpox never contracted smallpox. (Nowadays this sort of observation is frequently discounted as "anecdotal.") To make other people immune from smallpox, Jenner deliberately infected them with cowpox. He didn't know smallpox was caused by a virus. Pasteur would not propose his germ theory of disease until well into the next century.

Jenner just reasoned inductively from the evidence around him and thought up an ingenious way to save lives.

It's wise to recall that, much as our culture reveres science, when faced with different kinds of questions it routinely resorts to a totally different form of inquiry. I'm talking about the judicial system. Move the search for truth to a courtroom and the honest testimony of everyday people is welcomed, not dismissed as anecdotal. And the person who claims to have witnessed a crime—in contrast to a psychic event—is not automatically labeled as crazy or deluded.

The scientific method is fine as far as it goes. Such disciplines as biology and chemistry and most modern technology could scarcely exist without it. Thanks to our long-standing tradition of analytical, non-mystical thinking, workers in steel and plastics factories have no need to recite incantations, perform sacrifices, or even meditate before they cast their molten potions. But perhaps because too many decisions about how much is to be manufactured and what is to be done with it are made in a strictly left brain way, society ends up with too many "smart" bombs poised to destroy other people's bridges, too many hazardous, gas-guzzling sports utility vehicles, and an ever shrinking commitment to meeting basic human needs and supporting the achievement of higher goals. When we take it for granted that anything we can't examine in a laboratory, or do a controlled study on, or reduce to a mathematical formula is automatically not worthy of notice, we risk missing some of the most vital underpinnings of life.

Admittedly, many beliefs and practices of "primitives" and the unschooled look pretty bizarre to people brought up in the Western rationalist tradition. Sometimes a culture gap makes them sound more bizarre than they are. For instance, when I was doing research on the Zoroastrians, I ran across one scholar's reference to their purification rituals. One of these, he said, involved cleansing first with cow urine, then with sand, and finally with water. I blanched. *Cow urine? Cow urine for purification?*

Then I read a more thoughtful analysis of this very same ritual. As Mary Boyce pointed out in her book *The Zoroastrians,* cow urine is rich in ammonia, a pungent fluid widely used in household cleaning as well as for many industrial applications. The ancient Persians were pastoral nomads; they made their living crisscrossing arid lands with herds of cattle. For purification, Boyce said, they used what they had.

In Pietro di Donato's classic autobiographical novel of the Depression era, *Christ in Concrete*, immigrant Italian bricklayers demonstrate the same folk wisdom. When the 12-year-old protagonist's father is killed in a grotesque accident on a construction site, the boy, Paul, is forced to take his place as best he can. On his first day laying brick, he smashes his thumb with his trowel; scratchy brickdust and hot lime mortar eat into his hands. A fellow worker tells him, "Pee on your hands. . . . The pee contains nature's salt and heals quickly the bricklayer's finger." Then he binds Paul's wet hands with tape and tells the boy to keep them bandaged. At the end of his first grueling week, Paul feels tormented by his brutally aching back and joints—but his hands have healed.

Let's move on to something less indecorous. As a dedicated cook and diner, I can't resist mentioning a few examples of folk wisdom that relate to food. For centuries people have preserved meats by corning or smoking them. Both these processes produce cancer-causing nitrates—but the dangerous effects of these nitrates can be countered by vitamin C. If you're aware that both cabbage and tomatoes are fine sources of vitamin C, you've got to be struck by the way nitrate-heavy meats are traditionally served with their antidotes: corned beef and cabbage, hot dogs and sauerkraut, bacon and tomato, to name just a few. What Easterners call a "Western omelet" combines ham with chunks of bell peppers, another excellent source of vitamin C. If your local German restaurant doesn't serve sausages—most of which contain nitrates—with sauerkraut, they're likely to serve colorful sweet and sour red cabbage instead. Jewish delis traditionally supply cole slaw as a garnish for their overstuffed corned beef sandwiches. Healthy combinations like these abound in folk cuisine. Housewives with shamanistic insight figured these things out before the chemists did.

Shamans are experts on "other ways of knowing," their sources of information are paranormal, perhaps divine. Many of the substances we value for their healing qualities were first identified by shamans in Latin American rain forests or other remote places. In the recent best-seller, *Kitchen Table Wisdom,* Dr. Rachel Naomi Remen tells the story of a physician, the director of a neonatal unit, who, when a tiny baby appeared to be failing in spite of all her unit's best efforts, went down the hall to the hospital's chapel to collect herself before she told a young father that his son was going to die. After brief meditation, she had a strange thought—an impulse to treat the child with a drug not ordinarily used for the problems he had.

Ashamed to ask a nurse to inject such an unorthodox remedy, she administered it herself. Amazingly, the child recovered. Two years later the doctor heard that brand new research proved the remedy she used did indeed work with premature infants—but at the time she herself had used it, no such research was being discussed. Had she, like a shaman, sensed its efficacy by tapping into some paranormal source?

As we've seen, many people shrink from discussing their after-death contact experiences because they're fearful of being thought crazy, or because they don't want to sound superstitious and ignorant. Others don't dare give credence to their experiences *not* because they think they're illusions but because they've been taught by their religion to view them as coming from a satanic source.

Laura is the mortgage broker who for years worked with her husband, Dave, as a missionary for a fundamentalist church. Later, after Dave committed suicide, she sensed many ADCs with him. Here's how she felt about spirit survival and contact with the dead when she was a missionary.

> I would have thought what I sensed was a demon. That it wasn't Dave, it was just an imposter. That's what I was taught.

In Chapter 2 we heard from Katya about her psychic contact with her uncle at the moment of his death. The daughter of a minister, she told me also about a telepathic experience of hers which aroused an unexpected outburst from her father.

When I was about 16, I moved from Idaho to Oregon and left a very dear friend, a girlfriend that I would write daily. I had a chain I wore around my neck all the time. I had bought her a little "I Am a Presbyterian" thing, one for her and one for me, and I woke up as our clock in the hallway was chiming. I was yelling. I said, "Dad, something's happened to Barbara." And he said, "What do you mean?" And I said, "My chain just choked me and I know she's been hurt somewhere, something's terrible." And he said, "Don't listen to those kinds of things, that's of the devil," and he never spoke to me about it again.

The weird thing is he had never, ever mentioned the devil before in my entire growing up. His kind of liberal Presbyterians didn't talk about hell or damnation or the devil but this was something that evidently triggered something in him. Anyway about five days later, I hadn't heard from Barbara and I wanted to call her and of course I couldn't and I got a letter from her and she had been, that very night, on a ride with some kids out in the country and had been in a terrible accident. And it was exactly the same time that my chain squeezed my neck.

What in the Judeo-Christian tradition ever sired this fierce mistrust of contact through non-material routes? Now, I can't claim to be an expert on the Good Book. My religious roots are tangled at best. My mother, born into a non-observant Jewish family, lost her own mother when she was eight and soon came under the influence of a Protestant teacher whom she idolized. Then after she felt that she'd been cured of arthritis through faith, she became a devout Christian Scientist. Each day throughout much of my childhood she studied passages from her King James Bible along with passages written by the founder of Christian Science, Mary Baker Eddy. Often I borrowed her Bible to read it myself. Meanwhile my father and much older brother remained ardent atheists.

Bernice, the girl I thought of as my older sister—twelve years my senior—was in fact my mother's orphaned niece. For five and a half of her first six years—until my parents felt ready to bring her to live with them—she had lived in a devoutly Catholic home, kindly tended by three "old maid" schoolteacher sisters. Probably out of deference to Bernice's beginnings, I was taught to believe in Santa

Claus and was given presents at Christmas. Little wonder that, exposed to this mix of influences, I opted for what I viewed as the middle ground, agnosticism. But in recent years as my own faith in the divine and my interest in the afterlife have grown, I've delved into scholarly commentaries on the scriptures and I've interviewed members of the clergy far more knowledgeable than I.

Some of the uneasiness of clerics about paranormal contacts seems to stem from a confusion between visitations engineered by mediums and spontaneous experiences of the sort dealt with in this book. The Old and New Testaments are peppered with threatening references to intermediaries like that good-hearted "witch of Endor." In Exodus, Leviticus and Deuteronomy, the Israelites are told never to turn to mediums or wizards "to be defiled by them." Those who act as mediums face a fearful end. "A man or a woman who is a medium or a wizard shall be put to death; they shall be stoned with stones, their blood shall be upon them." Worst of all are said to be those who predict the future by consulting departed spirits. Nonetheless there's ample evidence in the Bible that the Israelites were familiar with neighboring peoples who trusted and relied on the guidance of sensitives and magicians of various sorts. Even among the Hebrews themselves, some such practices seem to have survived.

Curiously enough, there doesn't seem to be any Biblical injunction against gaining paranormal information from dreams— though this is a common route for after-death contact. In two Old Testament stories a Hebrew sage gains honor and advancement by interpreting his ruler's dream. (Unlike most of the after-death contacts described in this book, the dreams involved are thought to come directly from God rather than from departed mortals.) Joseph is released from a dungeon—freshly shaven and cleaned up for the occasion—to explain to Pharaoh that Egypt faces seven years of plenty which will be followed by seven of famine. (Genesis 41) Daniel describes to Nebuchadnezzer the troubling vision that the king has kept secret: a towering idol wrought of many metals that shattered before his eyes. Then he tells Nebuchadnezzer that it foretells the kingdoms that will follow his own. (Daniel 2)

In our own day, people who hesitate to tell a friend about an after-death contact experienced while awake, don't hesitate to say they've sensed a loved one's presence while asleep. The ten widows interviewed in Dr. Conant's 1992 study, reported in Chapter 1, described just such behavior in their bereavement groups.

It's probably still uncommon for people who've sensed ADCs to discuss them with their pastors or rabbis. Back in 1971, when a Welsh physician interviewed 293 widows and widowers, he found that although almost half of them had at some time sensed the presence of their dead spouse by some route other than dreams, none had ever volunteered this information to a doctor and only one had confided in a clergyman. When in 1999 I broached this subject to seven members of the clergy—Catholic, Protestant and Jewish—only two mentioned ever having been told of any such thing. The most forthcoming of the seven shared stories with me about the beliefs of a Chinese congregation he once served in the Far East.

The terror of demonic contacts suggested by Laura and Katya earlier in this chapter recalls an incisive observation made by Geddes MacGregor, writing in the *Encyclopedia of Religion*. MacGregor points out that confusion about the fate of the immortal soul after death has made the study of final matters such as death and judgment—"the least coherent aspect of the Christian theological tradition."

What becomes of the soul after death? Does it face immediate personal judgment and then move on to the destination its earthly behavior has merited: heaven, hell or some alternative place of punishment or instruction? Or must it sleep until the Final Judgment? *Fundamentalists who believe that it must indeed sleep, necessarily see spirit contacts as dangerous delusions that can only come from the devil.*

The apostle Paul promised resurrection—rebirth in a healthy body—at the second coming of Christ, "with the archangel's call and with the sound of God's trumpet," (I Thessalonians 4:16). Until that moment, most of the earliest Christians seem to have believed that the dead must sleep, totally out of reach. But it's wise to recall that Paul's audience believed that Jesus would return to them *during their lifetime on earth.* The next verse of Paul's letter makes that clear. "*We who are alive, who are left,* will be caught up in the clouds together with [the dead in Christ] to meet the Lord in the air...." Little wonder that some of those early Christian martyrs went singing to face the Roman lions. They thought of heaven as just around the corner. But as the centuries wore on and that final trumpet never did sound, the official Christian concept of resurrection was obliged to change.

Roman Catholics came to believe that there were saints already in heaven who intervened for and helped their fellow Christians on earth. They accepted a view of the afterlife that matched the words Jesus is said to have spoken to the thief crucified beside him, "Truly I say to you, today you will be with me in Paradise." [Luke 23:43] A story in the Apocrypha [2 Maccabees 7] reveals a similar belief in an immediate heavenly reward. A young man whose six brothers have just been brutally put to death for refusing to eat pork tells his tormenter, King Antiochus, "Our brothers, after enduring brief pain, have drunk of never-failing life."

Gradually the Catholics developed the notion of purgatory, an intermediate state which, like Paradise, had been suggested by some Jewish thinkers around the time of Christ. Until the 16th century, a certain amount of interplay between the living and the souls of at least some of the dead was taken for granted by virtually all Christians. But then Martin Luther—enraged by Church corruption with respect to pretended relics of saints and the selling of dispensations from time in purgatory—denied the existence of both saints and purgatory. Of course, Roman Catholics, Eastern Orthodox Christians—and Moslems as well—still endorse the veneration of saints.

Episcopalians occupy a middle ground. They retain belief in the Communion of Saints: spiritual union, variously defined, between holy persons on earth and saints, the Holy Trinity and angels in heaven. Nonetheless, the Reformation, as Renee Haynes has described it from a more strictly Protestant point of view, severed "the primeval threads of continuity between the living and the dead. The idea of purgatory, where they could be linked in prayer for one another was fading away ... and with it another idea, held among Christians quite certainly from the [fourth century] onwards, that *departed souls might sometimes come back unasked to comfort the bereaved or to set some matter straight.*" [Italics added.] It followed that "there was to be no more prayer to the saints, dead humans who in their holiness could still love and help living ones."

A tract issued by the Jehovah's Witnesses confronts this issue directly: "For his disobedience . . . Adam was sentenced to return to dust, to a state of nonexistence. . . . Yet someone may ask: 'Don't humans have an immortal soul that survives death?' Many have taught . . . that death is a doorway to another life. But that idea does not come from the Bible. . . . When the enemy death strikes, your grief can be great. . . . Yet, because you have confidence in the resurrection, your sorrow will not be unrelenting."

No matter what theologians, whatever their religious persuasion, have had to say about the spirits of the dead, ordinary people have continued to sense their presence. Each November, Mexicans—melding ancient Catholic observances with indigenous traditions—celebrate two Days of the Dead. They build home altars where they offer food and drink to the spirits of the deceased. They picnic in cemeteries, decorating graves with compazúchil flowers, round and yellow like the sun, then with the flowers' bright petals they trace a symbolic path outside their homes to lead the returning spirit to its altar.

The Dybbuk, one of the best known plays ever written in Yiddish, tells the story of a beautiful and pure young girl whose body is possessed by her dead fiance; his spirit cannot bear to part from her. *Webster's Third International Dictionary* defines "dybbuk" as "an evil spirit or the wandering soul of a dead person believed in Jewish folklore to enter the body of a man and control his actions until exorcised by a religious rite." Rites of exorcism, of course, are well known in Christian traditions as well.

The holiday that Americans call Halloween can be traced back to Samhain (pronounced "sa´win), a pagan celebration of the beginning of winter that takes for granted the existence of spirits. The ancient Celts thought that on the eve of Samhain and on Samhain itself, the barriers between the human world and the realm of the occult could be breached. The souls of the dead could visit the living while the living in their turn might penetrate the haunts of gods and supernatural creatures. No wonder witches took to their brooms that night! When Celtic peoples clung to this holiday even after they'd converted to Christianity, the British church tried to divert their attention from it by adding the Feast of All Saints to its calendar, setting it on the same date as Samhain. The eve of the festival was called Allhallows Eve, but its magical aspects won out over its saintly ones and in time it turned into that prankish event called Halloween.

As of late 1994, 90% of Americans said they believed that some sort of heaven exists. (It seems safe to say that most of these believers, untroubled by theological niceties, assumed that those lucky enough to get to heaven, arrived there soon after death.) Only 73% believed in hell, 72% believed in angels, and 65% believed in the Devil. When asked if people could hear from or communicate mentally with someone who had died, 28% said they believed and another 20% said they weren't sure.

Lots of people acknowledge some guarded belief in spirits in a casual, let's-have-fun-with-this sort of way. I'm all for fun but for me the thrilling part about looking at after-death communication is that there's loads of evidence for its reality through the ages. Towering figures like Swedenborg and Jung, Napoleon and Lincoln, have acknowledged having paranormal experiences of their own. But for the most part, there's a lingering taboo in our society against admitting that you've sensed anything of the sort.

It's high time that someone challenged that taboo in a serious, analytical way. Judging from the frequency with which religions around the world have come up with notions and observances that suggest occasional visits to the living by spirits, the odds are awfully strong that since time immemorial, contacts with the dead have been part of the human experience. Denying their reality threatens our mental health—and it's probably also dangerous to the planet.

Our modern world speeds heedlessly on, glittering and gleaming and crushing much in its path. Most of us have little time for meditation. We trade our time for the material wealth that our culture creates in abundance. Science as we know it enables the creation of this wealth. Nonetheless, so long as we deny the sacred and the numinous, the planet's fragile freight of life is in growing jeopardy.

6

After a Suicide

AT THE CLOSE OF CHAPTER 3, we heard from Laura whose husband, Dave, had committed suicide. Seven months after his death, she and her daughter had interlocking experiences of comforting contact with his spirit. But before then, she and others had received mixed messages from Dave. Soon after he died, Laura's daughter told her about a reassuring dream she'd just had.

Janie told me she saw daddy driving around in his car in our neighborhood and he was smiling and waving at her. She had the impression that he'd driven around five times. Now prior to his death, he was so depressed that he was also very paranoid. He wouldn't leave the house without someone else in the car. Janie didn't have a job at the time so she took care of him. So for her that he was driving around in his car without her and smiling was a big deal.

So then I said, "Do you know what the number five means? This is religious training that daddy and I have. The number five is the number of grace." I don't know where people come up with these things but that's what we were taught when we were missionaries for this evangelical Christian organization. Coming from that kind of perspective, suicide meant that you automatically went to hell so this thing about grace was a huge big deal.

So I was reassuring her, that was really exciting, and then I told her, "I just saw daddy too. I don't know if I was awake or asleep but it was so clear to me. He had this big beaming grin, which I haven't seen on his face in two or three years. This beautiful, pure, sunshining grin just beaming out of his eyes. And I had the distinct impression that he wanted me to know that he was okay." And then Steve's dream was that he and Dave were sailing in the sunset.

But a few weeks later, Laura sensed that something far more frightening might be happening to Dave.

I had this horrible dream. There was a grayish-brownish, a smog kind of mist and it was like Dave's body parts were dismembered and he was calling to me in a panicked, distressed kind of voice saying, "Laura, I'm stuck." That really freaked me out because at the time I believed it was either heaven or hell. I didn't believe in any netherworld or purgatory or anything like that so I told myself it was a nightmare and tried to push it out of my head. Still it frightened me, it stunned me. I didn't know what to make of it.

Then about a month or so later, I was talking with Dave's oldest sister. Rita's very Catholic. Definitely believes in purgatory, believes in praying the rosary and all that stuff. We were talking and she said, "Dave has appeared to me a lot of times." The first night he appeared, she woke up, she was laying on her side, and this man was standing fully clothed by her bed. She reached out to see that her husband was in the bed and he was. At the same time her eyes traveled up and she saw Dave's face. She said he was looking thoughtful and kind of sober and serious and imploring. Like he was trying to get her to think about something but she said, "I didn't know what he was trying to tell me, I just knew he was trying to tell me something." This was a couple of weeks after that nightmare that I had. And she said he had a key in his hand.

Well, that key, I thought that could mean a lot of things. It was significant to me that the way his face looked was like the way it might've looked when he was getting in the car. The last tool he used was that key. That was the implement of his death. [Dave chose to die of carbon monoxide poisoning.]

Rita reached out to touch him and, snap, he disappeared. She said it took about a month of these experiences before she called me. Three or four times a week he would just appear, that first time was the only time he ever looked right in her eyes. After that he would always be kind of looking off in the distance. He'd be standing there just thinking—sometimes really close by, sometimes farther away. She says it got to where she saw him in daytime.

Now Rita's a very spiritual woman, very religious, and this kind of thing has happened to her a lot. She finally decided she's not crazy, she just sees people after they've died. What she does in response is she prays for them. So she was telling me, "Laura, I really think Dave needs our prayers. I think he's stuck." And that word jumped into my head. I'd completely forgotten my nightmare but that word "stuck" jumped in my head and it really disturbed me.

I hung up the phone. It was about eleven o'clock at night and I went running up and down the hall, stopping and looking at pictures that I have of him in my hallway and going, "Are you okay?" Because I had this distinct impression that he was okay right after he had died. I was just absolutely baffled.

Somewhere along the line I met a woman that is a mystic. I called her and she said it's not uncommon for people who have died a violent death or an untimely death to be stuck in—I don't remember what she called it. Limbo or the bardo—maybe the astral plane. In Shakespearean plays, they called it the netherworld. You know, when spirits traipsing the earth are stuck between worlds and what not. Lots of cultures around the world have this same kind of belief.

Anyway, I began to realize that maybe, oh my goodness, Dave may be stuck. So I was talking with this mystic, Joene—I absolutely respect this woman and what she believes. And her mission on this planet at this time in her life is to be like an intercessor for people who are dying or have died. To help them to not be earthbound and to get them through to the light, or wherever it is they're supposed to go. We spent several hours discussing this and she agreed to go help Dave. She was tired that day but she said usually she would do this pretty late at night and she'd call me and let me know how things were going. My daughter had made an appointment too to see her for another reason.

Next day Janie goes to see her, she comes back in and she says, "Oh by the way, Joene says she got daddy through." I mean, I was like, "*What?*" The next day I go back, I talk with Joene and she tells me that she saw him, that he was afraid of what he had to do. He thought that where he had to go meant he was going to hell. So she had to make it clear to him that where he had to go was not hell but he had to deal with the things that he did wrong in this life. She was telling me stuff that just confirmed for me, oh yeah, this is Dave. That he didn't believe that God loved him enough to overlook his wrongs, his misdeeds, his bad choices and whatever. And she said, "What I did was I filled a hallway full of angels and love to draw him through so he'd know that this accounting he had to face would be done in an atmosphere of love and light and acceptance. Not hell." So she got him through.

Well, I waited a month after that experience, didn't have any more nightmares. Then I called Rita and I asked, "Have you seen Dave lately?" And she goes, "No, I haven't." And I said, "When's the last time you saw him?" And she says, "Oh, just a few days after I talked to you," and that made me feel he was really okay because that was when Joene got him through.

Laura's husband seems to have made his transition quickly. Was this because he was mentally ill when he took his own life? Or because he had been agonizing about his own worthlessness in the sight of God? I've collected several other upbeat stories of ADCs with the spirits of people who had taken their lives quite recently. Here's what Penny told me:

When I was in college I had a friend who committed suicide and that was very hard for all of us. We were all like, Why? When someone takes their life it's different from an accident or an illness. There was no sense of saying good-bye so when he came to me in dreams, it was like good-bye. He was carrying his bicycle, he always liked to bike, he was free and I felt a sense of closure. I woke up from that feeling very good and very strongly that he was at peace. I had these dreams shortly after he did this and I've never dreamed about him since.

Lucy is a retired school teacher and mother of three who, unlike most of my informants, has had only one paranormal experience in her life.

My father was the most important person in my life. He had had heart disease for ten years. He was a very stoic sort of man who never complained but then when he was 70 he had a stroke. His right side was paralyzed—and he'd always been a very independent person. The dependence that that created for him on other people was something he couldn't endure. About a week after he returned home from the nursing home, he killed himself. It was amazing that he managed to get out of bed into a wheelchair. This gun was kept in a place that was very high but he managed to reach it and wheel himself out onto the back porch—he was a very fastidious sort of person—and killed himself. He left me a very touching note.

No more than a week after his death when I awoke one morning, he was standing at the foot of my bed. It seemed so real, it didn't seem like a dream, it seemed like reality. He was dressed as he ordinarily did, an open shirt, trousers, looking serious, nothing unusual, he was a serious man. And he said, "Don't worry about me, I'm okay." He was reassuring me that everything was all right.

When Roderick was only 17, a friend of his, a few years older, committed suicide after the girl he loved jilted him.

I come from a very small town where there was a memorial tower for veterans. Very high, about three hundred, four hundred steps. People walk up to the top of the tower. Don't go if you have vertigo cause it's kind of queasy. But at the top there's a rim around it so you can't fall off. You'd have to make a real effort. And at night, they close it. There's a gate around it. But my friend broke in and climbed the stairs and he jumped off.

Well, three or four months later he came to me in a dream, smiling. And quite happy. I know that sounds very stereotypical but quite happy and looking very bright and very young. He was young, but he looked brighter and younger. And he just said, "I'm okay."

People talk about, you know, if you commit suicide, you're damned. That was not my experience with him. Maybe he had to do some explaining, maybe he had to do some sort of atonement, I don't know. But he certainly didn't look like he was in the fiery pits of hell.

Elmer was not an intimate friend of Marietta, but she knew him well as a fellow resident of a small island community. Soon after he took his own life, she had an odd series of experiences that culminated in a breakthrough similar to Laura's.

I had a finger that went kind of numb. It was like I couldn't feel blood in it and it was cold and very strange. I thought, "Well, maybe I should go to the doctor." That went on for a while.

We were building contractors so we were looking for a real estate agent to list our houses and we were interviewing some people. We were talking to this guy and we started talking about life and stuff and he said, "I've just gone to this very psychic person." He said her name was Mother Cher or something. For some reason, I felt really compelled to call her.

So I got her phone number from this gentleman and I called her and she started talking and then she said to me, "Are you having some numbness in one of your fingers?" Now, I tell you I almost fell off my chair. So I made an appointment with her. I went into her room, we sat and got quiet. Then she started to ask me, she said, "I'm picking up on a male and his name starts with E. Do you know anyone that's made their transition recently? They're trying to get in touch with you. And I'm like, "E, E, E?" And all of a sudden I said, "Elmer." Because he had just committed suicide.

And she said, "This man is calling out to you to have you help him make his transition." And I'm like, "Oh, fuck, this is just amazing to me." So she held my hand and we started praying and all of a sudden I had an energy go through me that was like a bolt of lightning! And it went through her and it went through me and she said, "He's through."

I'm not kidding, Sylvia, it was like a bolt of lightning. And it wasn't something that was hurtful. It was just . . . whoa! It went through both of us and she said, "He's through into the Light." And my finger, within an hour, it was absolutely fine.

R.J. is the gay man who reported two death coincidences in Chapter 2. When the AIDS epidemic started in the gay community, his "whole nursing career came into use because people would come to me with these stories about dying. And a lot of my friends died." One man who was dying of AIDS decided to take his own life.

He called before he was gonna do it and asked me, "What do you think about this?" I said, "If you want to do this, go ahead." He's in Seattle and I'm in Eugene and he calls me and says, "I'm gonna have my favorite friends over to dinner, have my favorite chocolate mousse cake. I've loaded my portion up with the proper recipe from the Hemlock Society and I'm going. I'll see you later."

Three weeks went by and I wasn't sure if it was successful but I didn't want to call. So I'm on my bike waiting to cross this busy street.

I'm looking at this white jeep turning the corner and here he is waving from the jeep—and he'd been dead three weeks.

R.J. has had numerous paranormal experiences. He shared many of his beliefs with me. Though he had encouraged his dying friend to take his own life, his strongest focus is on living fully.

The people I knew with AIDS in Hawaii, they had this whole drama going on, they had all these diseases. I used to get into these phenomenal conversations about what this was all about. What I started doing was trying to empower people to *live*. One of my friends, I said to him, "I love you dearly but I am so damn sick and tired of listening to you talk about dying. You are so negative that even this tree you're sitting under is dying. Why don't you try living?" I didn't see him after that. Four years later he came back and said, "Look, I still have it but I don't even acknowledge it. I gotta give you credit, you set me right."

I've just had a conversation with a young woman whose husband died suddenly a week ago. She's totally distraught, needless to say, because they believed they had come together as two halves of one spirit. She said to me, "Do you think he misses me?" I said, "Darling, I've got bad news for you. He's not even thinking of you." She's talking about how she wants to take her own life to be with him. I said, "Let me tell you something. If you take your life, unless you take your life to go *toward* something, you're gonna go and you're gonna see him but my mental picture of this is that there'll be a thick glass wall between you and him for eternity and it'll be worse than any hell you can imagine."

Do some people who kill themselves have to endure long punishment after? Two women reported brief, cryptic ADCs that came to them many years after a suicide. Jan is a trim, chic person who works as a human resource manager. Some years after her former college roommate killed herself, Jan sensed contact with her.

We had lost touch with one another. We were living in different states and I had the opportunity to come visit her in the course of a trip I was going to take, so I wrote her a letter, told her I'd like to see her, and didn't hear back from her. I was pretty disappointed. Then I got a letter from her parents telling me she'd committed suicide. I wrote them back and told them how sorry I was and said that I certainly hoped it was *not* a suicide but just a mistake. Because she used to take a *lot* of medication. But I never heard back.

Some years later—it's not like I'd been thinking of her but she came to me in a dream and told me she was okay. She was sitting on the hood of a car, it was a sunny day, and I was putting money in a parking meter and she said, "I just wanted to tell you I'm okay." She looked just the same as I had always known her. In this dream, I knew she was dead so I said, "Wait a minute, wait a minute, I have to put money in this meter if I don't want to get a ticket but I want to talk to you!" I was thinking, wait a minute! Did you really commit suicide? She said, "No, I don't have time, but I just want you to know that I'm okay." And when I finished putting the money in the meter and turned around, she was gone. When I woke up I remember feeling just so perplexed. And yet I thought wow, this is kind of neat—now I know she's fine.

Christina is a cheerful, independent-minded woman who has had many kinds of paranormal experiences, some very detailed and informative. One of her most slight and subtle involved a relative who took her own life some twenty years before.

I was at the dentist's office—and suddenly I smelled her perfume. It was my Aunt Judy, who committed suicide. It couldn't have just been another patient with that perfume on. I knew it was her—but I don't know why she was there with me.

Denise is a bouncy, pretty woman who wore a Star of David to our interview. She's proud of her Russian Jewish roots but doesn't practice any organized religion and has been married to two non-Jews. Her ex-husband, Rick, was a logger. He killed himself ten years before our interview, then repeatedly made his presence known in unwelcome ways to her and their daughter.

We'd been divorced seven years when he shot himself but in this life he never left me alone anyway. He kind of like hounded me, he didn't stalk me. He'd lost his mother years before that. He was two years older than me but I became his caretaker. He was so needy, so dependent. One day it hit me what I was really doing and I didn't want to care for him anymore. When we were divorced, he would bring women over for me to check out for him. I guess it meant a lot to him if I liked her.

He lived with a lot of guilt, not coming to terms with things that he did wrong. Not being the son that he wished he was to his mother. Not being the son to his father. Not being the husband to me, not being the father, because of his alcohol and binges. And prior to that, he'd been in Vietnam. He got into heroin there when he was seventeen—just seventeen years old!

He just got off on the wrong track, he had a hard life. I had two children from before that he loved as his own. He never was physically abusive at all, it was the mental abuse on our family. When we were divorced, he was continually making promises to his daughter and breaking them. I'd tell him, "Don't make promises, then you won't break them!" He never paid support, never visited her regularly. Finally he told my daughter he'd be there for Thanksgiving and he didn't show up. It was four days after that that he killed himself. He was a hunter, he shot himself, he left a note. Ugh. He said my daughter would be better off. That was ten years ago and she's still having problems with it.

Anyhow, three days after he passed over, I had a dream. I was walking down a dark hall with doors on each side of the hallway. Now Rick was a logger so he was a real strong man. I just felt like someone came out a door and grabbed me from behind and I was like, "Is that you? I *know* it's you." And then I woke up and I said, "Oh, he came to me. He's letting me know he's here." What a way! So from then on it was continual, in dreams. One time I woke up when I'd been dreaming about him and there he was sitting at the end of the bed. I was awake and there he was sitting at the foot of the bed—and then he just disappeared. It was, oh my god! He looked the same. He was just staring at me and then he disappeared.

So then at work, I'd be walking down the hall and I'd hear his voice—he had a real rough voice—and I heard my name being yelled out. And I'd turn around and stop—and no one was there. Then I'd be sitting at my desk in my office at the TV station and all of a sudden that sense came on me that he was right there in my face somewhere. I'd say, "What do you want?" I'd say it out loud. I was alone in my office, no one could hear. For twelve years I was operations coordinator for programming there. This was all before I met my new husband.

Then my daughter, she kept thinking she heard Rick. One day in school—she was ten by now, it was almost a year since he died—she thought she heard him yell her name. She turned around and saw him sitting in a desk. She got so scared, she started screaming, running out of the room. She went to the counselor.

Well, thank goodness, this counselor at her school, he'd had experiences with his granddaughter who died. So at least he didn't say my daughter's going crazy. I was grateful 'cause I told him right in the beginning, "I believe my daughter. I don't know what you believe in." And he goes, "Oh, no, no." And he explained his story. He said his daughter-in-law was a channeler. And he said to me, "If it's too much and your daughter's scared, you can ask him to go away."

So we did. Six months—nothing! It was strange, not feeling him anymore or dreaming about him. But at about six-ish months, I had a dream that he was walking in front. My view was like I was looking down on our house from above and I can see him walking on the sidewalk in a trench coat. He was walking along the sidewalk and trying to peek in the windows, trying to see if he could get a glimpse of us, wanting to come in.

I asked her what was special about her dreams of Rick. How did they differ from ordinary dreams? Paranormal dreams are often described as "vivid." In Chapter 12 I talk about this more. Here's how Denise responded to me.

It's kind of a cliché maybe, but everything with him in it was so real. I woke up feeling I was in his world or something. Like we came and met in a different area. I woke up just *knowing*. The brain isn't thinking, it's the intuition. I'd wake up knowing that was him coming to me.

So then I meet my now-husband. We date a while, then he moves in, then we get married. One time I wake up crying. In my dream Rick was laying in bed with my husband and I and it just scared me to death. I woke up and I grabbed my husband, I'm whimpering and I'm wailing. Three times my husband and I are asleep in the bed with the light out. We had no kids at home anymore, they're all gone. And three different times, the light is on in the middle of the night. We wake up and my husband goes, "Did you turn the light on?" "No!" I tell him. You wake up and it's light in your room and it's so odd, it's too much. When Rick comes, it's not like an angel and soothing. He just never will leave me alone.

For Rick's transition to the afterlife, his suicide seems to have been the least of his problems! His is a classic case of the spirit who cannot acknowledge that he's dead, cannot break his earthly ties. This chapter's last story is far more romantic. It's a tale of a soulmate lost, then found—then lost and found again.

When Gary was in his twenties, he owned two tractor-trailer rigs and was a long distance hauler. He fell in love with Susan, more deeply in love than he'd ever been before. She accepted his invitation to ride along with him for one trip, then for two years they were virtually inseparable, traveling together from one end of the country to the other. Gary recalled those years as incomparably sweet. Cramped together in a little semi, he said, they didn't need to talk. They could sense each other's feelings and have long conversations without ever speaking a word. Then Susan got pregnant. Soon she couldn't endure their hard life on the road. He urged her to marry him but she refused. Back home she fell in with the wrong sort of people, got hooked on drugs, and her relationship with Gary fell apart.

> Every time I'd come home she'd look more pale, more out of it, not having that pregnant glow. I started to get really concerned but luckily it was a normal pregnancy. My daughter's a very healthy girl. I was hoping that having our daughter would kind of pull us back together but it didn't work. So I figured the proper thing for me to do was to become the custodial parent because of my income. Susan was obviously out of control of her life. So I sold my trucks to pay for my lawyers. After about eight months of nonstop court battles, the courts awarded me custody, then Susan disappeared before my daughter was a year old.
>
> She stayed gone for ten or eleven years. One day she came back, just showed up out of the clear blue and it was absolutely amazing. She looked healthy again, like the girl I fell in love with all those years ago. Her attitude was better, her mental state was better. Unfortunately in the process she'd picked up a husband and two other

children so I figured, well, that closed the door on that. But we used to have long talks in the park and on the phone—about how she felt the same way I did, that instead of her being married to someone else it should have been us. Only now she had two more children. So it's not like you can just pick up and follow where your instincts are. But for about a year we got incredibly close.

Unfortunately she had a relapse and fell back into drugs again which I guess happens with addicts. One night her husband called me up in the middle of the night and told me that Sue took her life. So here my daughter was just getting to know her mother that was gone all those years and now I had to tell my daughter. The loss was just absolutely incredible for my daughter and me.

So for maybe two years after that, I kind of let the feeling of loss turn down to a slow boil. Every once in a while I'd kind of catch her out of the corner of my eye, see her dancing off on the side of my field of vision. I kind of expected that, it was easy to pass that off. I'd go out to where she's interred and talk to her every once in a while. Never got an answer, just a feeling of comfort. Felt better but I never got anything resolved.

Then about a year ago I had minor surgery. I picked up an infection, they had me pretty severely medicated, and I had a dream where for some reason I woke up in an absolute terror. I don't know what brought it on. In this dream, the door of the room I was in opened up and *Sue* came walking in and sat down on the edge of the bed, hugged me, whispered things to me and told me everything was gonna be all right. Told me to lay back down and go to sleep. And I did. In my dream I did and when I woke up it was like I could almost smell her scent, like she just left the room for a second to get something. Does that make sense?

She had this particular perfume that she loved to wear—it's not one you find a lot of people wearing. I hadn't smelled it for a long time but when I woke up it was like just the hint of it, like a tease of a scent in the air but it was enough for me to pick up right away and to *me* it was incredibly *real*. When she was in my dream it was so lifelike. I could feel her body heat when she was holding me, feel her hair and stuff. She was just holding me and comforting me and then just kind of laid me down, told me to go to sleep, and I wake up literally expecting to see her sitting there at the foot of the bed. And I thought I should feel glad, because I was able to see her again, it was so realistic. It was hard to believe it was a dream but it really just opened that sense of loss again. It was like getting a taste of what you want all your life and then not being able to have it again. Then this past Wednesday I had an experience that just floored me. I had to actually leave work.

The place where I work now, we do public opinion polls and surveys and we were doing this poll in San Jose. I've driven through San Jose but I don't know anybody there and it's all blind surveys, we don't know who we're calling or whatever. So I'm talking to this lady. I have no idea who she is, she has no idea who I am. And about halfway through the survey she goes, "Your name's Gary, right?" I go yes—maybe I introduced myself at the beginning of the survey. She goes, "You're 44, aren't you?"* Yeah—well, maybe she can guess from my voice or whatever. She goes, "I'm gonna tell you something, you may think I'm absolutely crazy but I have a message for you."

Okay, I figure, this is where they start telling me I'm taking up too much of their time and hang up. She goes, "There's a lady named Sue or Susan, do you know her?" "Well," I said, "I did know a Susan." She goes, "Okay, I wanna tell you, I'm a psychic. I work with police departments and whatever. You may think I'm crazy but Sue has a message for you. She says that she watches over you while you sleep"—which made me think right away of the deal in the hospital—"and she wants you to know that when she left, the air was burning but she's flying in cool air now." And what really hit close to home was the way Sue took her life, she locked herself in the garage with the car running and got all that hot gases and everything in there. So I just stopped the survey right away. I'm thinking this can't be happening. I'm peppering this lady with questions. "Did she say anything else?" I've got tears going down my face. People around me are looking at me like, Jesus, Gary, you've got a bad one there. She goes, "Sue wants you to let go, just let go."

So I'm telling this lady, "So how do I do that? That was my destiny to be with that lady and nobody can convince me otherwise, that was the lady I was supposed to be with." So she's telling me all these things. "Go home, light a white candle...." Things like that.

---

* If Gary's story sounds improbable, here's another that matches it. A Scotsman from a family of psychics was quoted as saying about his mother, "if she never met you in her life before, she could tell ye your name and age an everything aboot ye." [B. McDermitt. (1986) 'Stanley Robertson.' *Tocher* 40: 170-186.]

"Sue wants you to know that she'll always be watching over you but to let her go."

I've known other people who thought they were psychics but they only talked in broad generalities. This lady got Sue's name right from the start and then the deal about the hot air, flying through hot air. I never gave much thought to ghosts, whatever, but now, now I do. Everything is so layered on everything. You know, first Sue, then the psychic, and two days later I see your little ad in the paper. It's all leading somewhere.

I couldn't help but agree. He seemed to have been led to me for a very special purpose.

Gary was the seventh person I interviewed. The story he told me bore an eerie resemblance to a story I'd heard earlier from Beverly, whose death coincidence is cited in Chapter 2. The same year that Gary had lost his soulmate, Beverly—a little younger than Gary, and like Gary, an attractive, vivid person—had lost her beloved husband of nineteen years to an unexpected illness. Like Gary, she had clung faithfully to the memory of her lost love, refusing to seek a new partner. In dreams, she'd seen her late husband and smelled his favorite scent, Royal Copenhagen, while he told that he loved her and that he was okay but that she had to get on with her life. Once she awakened from a dream of him to feel his scent still on her. This is how she described that experience:

> I hadn't had any of his stuff around for the last couple of years but when I woke up I could smell Royal Copenhagen all over my body. I could *smell* it on me so I knew we had met someplace. Although it appeared to be in the physical realm, I knew it wasn't. I knew I was with *him*.

Maybe, I thought, the universe meant for these two loyal, lonely people to meet each other. And maybe it was my job to help make this happen. So I told Gary something of what Beverly had said, asked him if he'd be willing to phone Beverly, then asked Beverly if she'd mind if Gary phoned her. Their first phone conversation lasted two hours. Soon they discovered more similarities. Each had a teenage daughter; both daughters had the same, uncommon first name. And Beverly's own middle name was Susan. I started wondering when I'd get a chance to attend their wedding!

So far, no such luck. They saw each other for months but when last heard from, they'd broken up. Probably their friendship was just an important first step toward their letting go and getting on with their lives.

In the next chapter we'll hear from other people who, like Beverly and Gary, have learned from scents and even subtler signs that loved ones have come to visit them.

7

Subtle Contacts—Smells and a Sense of Closeness

Dᴏᴇꜱ ᴀɴʏᴛʜɪɴɢ ʙʀɪɴɢ ʙᴀᴄᴋ ᴀ ʀᴜꜱʜ ᴏꜰ ᴍᴇᴍᴏʀɪᴇꜱ more vividly than a familiar smell? When I was five, I visited relatives in Vermont. We never again visited them there but every now and then, many decades later, I catch a whiff of an odd odor that lurks in damp, dark old wooden structures and I'm back exploring their storage shed. I crush in my fingers the sweet smelling seeds of one particular weed and once again I'm playing with my cousins; we're throwing a fragrant rain of seeds at each other.

Almost a third of my informants reported paranormal experiences that involved scents. Men seem to be particularly aware of women's perfumes. Nancy was not simply Joe's mother-in-law—he considered her a dear friend.

> She died of breast cancer, complications from breast cancer. I was certainly very close to her and my wife was devastated by her loss. There are many, many cases when my wife or I are under stress and the room will suddenly be filled with her favorite perfume. It's just an incredibly peaceful thing, it reminds us of her. It's almost as though she's there looking over our shoulder and saying it's okay, everything's fine.

Tom's first wife died two years before I interviewed him. Though their marriage ended in divorce, he still remembers her fondly.

When I visit her grave site, the air can be completely dead but when I go down there, there's always a gentle breeze and I can smell the perfume that she wore. She always walks me back to the gate because I've gotten in my car and I can smell her perfume. I've looked around for flowers thinking that their fragrance would just have blown in the window but there's no flowers there so I know it's her.

Jerry grew up with an abusive, alcoholic father and no mother in the home. He had no religious training and no belief in the paranormal. Now a longtime Quaker, he's deeply spiritual and devoted to the way of peace but during World War II, as a 17 year-old marine, he experienced a battlefield conversion in two stages. He told me this story with bursts of rueful laughter and a satiric sense of the inappropriateness of the racial epithet that he—and other marines at the time—had used.

My first night in combat on Iwo Jima, I climbed into a shell hole to defend our company and there were six corpses in there, four Japanese and two Marines. The "gooks" had been there for some time and they were rotting and the flies were coming out of their mouths and their skin was purple and cracked, the Marines however had been freshly killed.

Every twelve seconds in combat the mortars behind you shoot off flares and they go up and break with a pop and they come down with little parachutes on 'em so you can see what's going on. So I could see the "gooks" and the dead Marines and all of a sudden I heard all this jabbering down the cliff in front of us and the Japanese were getting ready to banzai. It really was too much for me and I started crying and I promised God—it sounds so silly—if you'll get me out of this, I'll go to church every Sunday the rest of my life. That's all I knew.

And lo and behold, a breeze came up from the sea and this was the most calming, the most tranquilizing, the most peaceful experience I've probably ever had in my life. It just told me that everything would be fine. Don't worry about things. Had no problems the rest of the operation and about a week later, we were on the point in combat. The point in combat is in the morning where you have to send people out to find where the enemy is so you can attack 'em. So out we go, about six of us, and all of a sudden we get pinned down by the Japanese. They've almost surrounded us and they kept firing everything into us and we're in this hole and we have to find someone to relieve us to get these people off our back.

All of a sudden the radio quits, so the lieutenant writes out a note and he says to me, "Well, here are our coordinates. Go back and give this to the artillery." Well, there's machine guns blasting away and mortars blasting away. Everything is blasting away and I think I'm dead. So I start off and of course we'd been up all night and after about fifty feet, I was just too tired. I said the hell with it. Kill me. And like a giant hand—I can only describe it as a giant hand—was put up and just protected me. Everything went by me, nothing hit me. Bullets flying every place, didn't bother me at all. So, you know, I didn't go to church every Sunday but I became a believer in God and a believer in people.

When Jerry came back from the war, he had a scent experience that awakened his belief in spirit survival. He'd been living in New York City, some distance from his New England hometown. Years before, his father had remarried and his new wife's mother—Jerry's step-grandmother—had come to live with them.

Boy, she was something else. She'd invite me up to her room and break out cigars and we'd sit there smoking cigars. A year after she died, I came up to visit 'em and I slept in her old room and she awakened me. She awakened me because she had a very peculiar type of perfume. I'd never smelled that smell on anyone else. And she would trail it right by the bed and wake me up. She woke me up three times that night with that smell. And then as soon as I woke up, it would go away. It was almost like she walked by deliberately, went Whoof, and kept going. Well, by then I'd been with death a long time, and spiritual and stuff so it didn't bother me but I called her and I'd say, "Grammy, are you there?" And I would get no reply, of course. Fall asleep and she'd come by and do it again. I didn't know what to make of it but she sure gave me a clue. I *knew* there was another life because that night she kept coming, waking me up.

In the previous chapter, Christina told us about briefly smelling her Aunt Judy's perfume some twenty years after her death. After Barbara's mother died, the scent of her perfume became Barbara's constant companion.

Mother usually wore Crêpe de Chine. And I thought it was my imagination. I could not get that smell out of my nose for five or six months after she died. That was all I smelled. I had the last bottle that she had. I'd thrown it in my underwear drawer, so I thought, "Maybe that's what it is." But it was almost empty. I moved it and put it someplace else and the scent just got stronger. She wore it her whole life. It's an old scent.

One New Year's Eve, when Cindy was at a small family gathering, she and two relatives smelled the kind of cigarette her grandmother used to smoke. But that was just the beginning of their contact experience that night.

My dad was out of the country then, so my husband and I were spending the holiday with my mom in their house. We were just sitting there having liqueurs—and I don't really care for liqueurs too much. But we had our three little glasses. They had a love seat against one wall and another love seat against the next wall and this big round coffee table was in between. My glass was a little bit further back, and then my mom's was on her side.

So we're sitting there, and all of sudden there is an incredible smell of cigarette. And neither of my parents smoke. My mom's mom smoked and she used to live with us when I was a child—she died when I was 15. So all of a sudden there is this incredible smell. She smoked a Canadian cigarette, a real distinctive smell. My mom and I just kind of looked at each other and then she said something like, "Can you smell smoke?" And I'm like, "Yeah." Even my husband could smell it. And he goes, "Well, where's that coming from?" So he looked around to make sure there wasn't anybody outside or anything, and he couldn't see anybody. So it was like somebody had been smoking and then left the room. So we're like, "Okay, that was kind of freaky."

So just a little bit later we were talking about how much that smelled like my grandmother's cigarettes and the weirdest thing happened to my liqueur glass. I had mine set further back than my husband's because he kept handing me his and I wasn't really drinking that much. So suddenly my liqueur glass went from about the middle of the table to the *front* of the table and fell off on the floor. And both the other glasses are just sitting there. There was just this dead silence and we all looked at each other. Me and my husband at the same time, we got up and went, "Well, gotta go now." *[Laughs]* And my mom says, "You sit down right now because that's pretty spooky. No one's leaving till I say they're leaving." *[Laughs]*

Eileen e-mailed me a similar story.

My late husband had been a smoker since serving in the Coast Guard. He tried many times over the years to stop smoking but was never able to do so for long. I am allergic to tobacco smoke so he usually went outdoors to have a cigarette. One evening last week as I sat at the computer, I smelled a strong odor of cigarette smoke. I was alone in the house and thought it was really odd but disregarded it. It then became very strong and I began having serious trouble breathing, so could no longer pass it off as imagination. Then it passed as suddenly as it started.

On thinking about it later, I could just imagine him thinking, "What could I do to convince Eileen that I am here in the room with her?" That particular choice would be typical of him! I was reminded of it yesterday when a member of my bereavement support group mentioned that she experienced a strong odor of her husband, who died recently, in their room.

On several occasions, Charlie and his son Don smelled odors they associated with Charlie's late father.

My son and I were in my office. There's a lot of stuff there from my father's house. I was sitting down and he was standing up, and he says, "I smell Grandpa!" And I said, "Yeah, I do too." It was like right at that moment we shared that experience, smelling his body odor as if he were there. Now you could say it's because my dad's things are there but we don't smell it all the time. It's not like we pulled his shoes out or something. There've been other times when Don said, "I can smell Grandpa in that room." It's happened to him more than once. One time within the last year I smelled my dad's cologne, this French Pinaud, a very distinctive smell, and I know I did not bring a bottle back from his house. He had one open bottle at his house when he died, but I didn't bring it back here.

Like Charlie, Penny has sensed more than one smell she associates with her father. One is what she called his "work clothes smell."

> I can remember his smell, I always feel it on my left side, I don't know why. He was a mechanic so he had a kind of oily quality.

Her mother recalled smelling the same scent at times.

> Once in a great while, if I'm doing something outside and I come in, I can almost smell his smell. Yeah, like he'd been there in the house after he'd been working on his car.

Penny used to live in the upstate New York region where, in the nineteenth century, Spiritualism began. For a time she attended "circles," seances where she studied to be a medium. Her father's spirit brought gifts to her there.

> He would come and once he brought me flowers. The smell was so intense that you could just feel the presence. After class he was still with me. I can remember sitting down in the parking lot because I was getting kind of heady. He would come and I can remember different messages that he would give my classmates to share with me. Like "Remind her about her drawings." I used to draw quite a lot as a child and he was showing my classmates these pictures that I would draw so they could validate them for me.
>
> It's very common for my father to come to me in my dreams, even still. I think that's because it's a purer channel. Our lives are so busy during the day but somehow in the sleep state we can be more open. I smell things, like I could smell the flowers that he gave me. It's like this beautiful bouquet.

Sometimes Elise works as a medium.

> When I work as a medium very often I will get scents. That's how spirits identify themselves. I will smell biscuits or something baking and it will be somebody's grandmother. Once I smelled cabbage rolls

and I hate cabbage but I explained it, I'm smelling this. And the young man who was sitting with me said, "Oh, my grandmother made the best stuffed cabbage." But more often the scents I get would be a rose or lilac or something like that.

Even more subtle than smelling a scent is sensing that in some indefinable way the spirit of a loved one has come to visit. They may come during vivid dreams or in waking moments. Two young women whom I interviewed had sensed dream contacts with great-grandparents. Here's what Spring experienced—and how it affected others in the family.

My great-grandmother died when I was in high school and a few years later I had a dream that I came home and turned on the answering machine and she was on the phone saying, "This is Nana. I just wanna say I'm thinking about you and make sure you're okay." I didn't think all that much about it at the time. I just thought that's an interesting way for her to get in touch with me. I really believe that's just what she did. So anyway, I told my dad and he told his father. Then my grandfather asked me about it. He said, "I heard you had this dream." I never expected him to think that anything like that was real but it was his mom. . . . He put some credence in it which I thought was great.

Carol reported contacts with a pair of her great-grandparents.

My mom's mother's parents died when I was eight and then ten years old and I remember them quite vividly. They come to me in dreams. They were great people. In fact, I have their wedding rings, my grandmother gave them to me. Mostly it's my great-grandmother. I took her Hebrew name and her mother's to become my Hebrew name because when I was born I wasn't given one. Sometimes I have dreams about her and my great-grandfather but they're not necessarily coming to me. Sometimes there are dreams where she comes to me and says hello. They're nice.

After a long career as a nurse, Roni switched professions to one better suited to her artistic talents. She now runs her own successful small business, creating dazzling costumes—sometimes for leading rock and operatic performers. When she was in her twenties, she lived for five years with Len, the man she calls the love of her life. Then they parted. Eventually each married somebody else, decades later both were widowed. Two years before I interviewed her, Roni and Len came together again—but after four months of delight in each other, Len died in Roni's arms of a heart attack.

He died in my bedroom. After he died for almost a month there was this shadow on the ceiling that never was there before. It was there during the daytime, it was there at night, it was always there. Even in the pitch dark, it was there. I'd look up at it and I'd talk to it. Then after a month, it went away.

I dream about him at least two or three times a week. He had the most stressful life. I had a dream about him one time. I was being held prisoner, I was being tortured and he came through a window to rescue me. We went into this little tiny plane. It was like a cartoon plane with people sitting on top, and then all of a sudden, he drove the plane right into a flower. And he says, "Now I'm free, now I'm safe and no one can hurt me anymore." It was astounding. It was like he was telling me, "Yah, now I'm okay. I couldn't live any longer. I was in too much emotional pain."

Sometimes I'll wake up after I've had a dream about him, in that period of time when you're not asleep and not awake and not cognizant and I'll wake up and I'll be saying, "Len, don't go yet, don't go. I want more time." That happens a lot. And then I'll look around and I'll know that I'm awake now. But I can feel his presence still. Sometimes I'll wake up and I can feel it all over. Inside of me. And like a hug. If I wake up and it's been one of those loving kind of dreams, I'll just feel so good and I'll feel his touch. That to me is the best.

Marti is a third generation Unitarian who grew up with no belief in an afterlife. When she was in her twenties, about to start graduate study in social work, and the mother of two small sons, her husband died. Soon she started experiencing contacts of various sorts with her late husband, some when she was awake, others when she was sleeping.

When I would dream of him, some of the dreams had a very special quality. Some of them were just junk dreams, unfinished business kind of dreams, and then there were others where I began to realize he made contact. There've been a couple of dreams where it's almost like seeing him across a crowded room. Not having actual contact with him but just kind of knowing he's there. Once he was there physically. I was in bed trying to sleep, half asleep, half awake, and it was like . . . you know when couples lie in bed in spoon position, that was what it was like and it was also highly comforting because that was a highly stressful time in my life.

Once I heard his voice—he said, "I love you." That was stunning. The time he said he loved me, that was when I was pondering a decision to leave where I'd been living and I was getting a lot of flak from people that didn't want me to. He was there to tell me I was on the right track. It was wonderful.

There was a period earlier when, when he came, I would get thrown back into some relatively deep grief. For many years now, when he makes contact basically it's like an old *friend* and it's lovely and thanks for calling.

One of Marti's sons also has sometimes sensed contact with his father. A handsome, well-built man in his early thirties, he works as a stone and brick mason.

My father died when I was eight. I really do feel that on occasions my father has been with me. Very often in the woods, backpacking and stuff. He liked to hike.

The first time, I was 18 or 19 and I was backpacking with a friend of mine. We had gone over a pass that didn't have a trail on it. We were kind of horsing around up on top and my friend turned his ankle pretty bad. He was gimping around, didn't feel like he could hike with his pack all the way down so things turned kind of serious. What we decided to do was I was gonna hike down with his pack and then come back up and get my stuff. He felt he could walk but he couldn't carry his pack. So anyway I got down, dropped the pack off, hiked back up—and it was an incredibly beautiful spot. Mount Shasta was off to my west, some thunderstorms over there. I sat down and I really felt my dad was with me.

I never physically saw him, I could feel his air. I wasn't getting any telepathic messages, just a feeling that he was in my presence.

That was ten or eleven years after he passed away. I got very emotional. Broke down and cried for five or ten minutes. I guess I was releasing a lot of built up things about him I hadn't thought about for a while. It really shook me up but it was great to feel like he was around.

For a time, both Sharon* and her husband served in the Naval Reserves. After her husband was killed in the crash of a Navy plane, his squadron commander offered to supply a plane from which she could scatter his ashes.

My husband was a sky person, he really loved the air so I said it would be great if I could get somebody to take me up in a little plane and scatter them up at Puget Sound because that's where the base was. So the squadron commander said, "Oh, we can arrange that. Who would you like to come along?" And I said just some of the people that were close, just the crew and me and a couple friends.

Well, they took one of our big transport planes, hundred passenger things, and I got my choice of crew and I picked my people that I really liked a lot. They said they would depressurize me, go down below 10,000 feet and stream a window open and I could dump him myself—that was kind of neat. It cost them thousands of dollars to bring this bird up in the air but that's what they did. And it was really, really stressful. A lot of emotion. I had my two friends sitting in the back of the plane with me. I had my flight engineer and my pilot and co-pilot and navigator up front. They were close to Ben so I chose them as a crew.

So I did the ashes out the window and it really upset me. I can remember I was in tears and I was sitting there and the guys just walked up and kind of touched me in a reassuring kind of way and walked away. But then, when there was *nobody, no one* sitting behind me, I felt a squeeze on my shoulder. Just this squeeze. It wasn't a spoken thing, it was in my head that said, "It's okay now, it's done." It was like all the tension lifted. I was no longer upset. I sat there and just kind of looked around as if, you know, who did that? Then I just sat there and let it kind of wash and I realized that it just had to be

---

*This is the second interviewee named Sharon who is quoted in this book. The other Sharon was interviewed along with her daughter, Penny.

something other than my emotions because I was not looking for it. It was a totally unexpected event.

So I sat there for a while, kind of mellowed out again, and that made the decision for me. I had the option of getting back out even though I had signed up for two years. They gave me the option of resigning the commission and going back out of the service. So I went up and plunked my shoulders down on the flight engineer's shoulders. They all looked around and gave me a "Hi, there." I said, "Well, I've decided what I want to do about your Man's Navy." They always called it their "Man's Navy." I said, "I'm gonna stay in and I'm gonna be the best damn load master and flight attendant you have." The guys all cheered and said, "Yeah, great!" It was fine. It was a tremendous relief.

Unfortunately, some contact experiences aren't comforting at all. When Roni's mother was alive, their relationship was dismal. The woman was psychotic. When Roni was a child, her mother often brutally beat her. After she died, for a couple of years Roni had an eerie sense that her mother's spirit was haunting her basement.

It was horrible because I'd be down in the basement and I *knew* she was there. I'd be washing clothes and all of a sudden I'd turn round real fast and say, Jesus fucking Christ, will you please . . . why are you tormenting me?

It wasn't in a loving, calm sense that my mother came to me. Whenever she came, all I felt was pure fright. It was the same feeling that I had all my life with her so in death it continued. When she was alive, my mother would come into a room sometimes, even when she was in a good mood, and she still gave me a fright and I couldn't help it.

My mother died when I was in my early forties. I got to the point where one day I said to her, "Mom, I'll let it all go. You don't have to keep coming back to me to ask me forgiveness or anything. It's okay." I knew that's what it was all about. It was that she just felt so bad about the past. I did a little ritual: salt, candles, everything, down in the basement—cause I practice paganism to a certain extent. Then one Mother's Day, I woke up, I went out on my deck and I just shouted, "Happy Mother's Day!" And I don't hate her anymore.

Three women had deeply moving sense of presence experiences that involved reconciliations with their fathers. Chris used to travel a lot on business.

> My father passed away nine years ago and probably two or three years after that I was in a hotel room in Denver and *he was there.* I don't know how else to say it except I could just feel his presence. I was not expecting it at all. I had the television on, I don't remember what I was watching, but all of a sudden he was there.
>
> When I was younger we were very, very close. Then over a period of time he became an alcoholic and some of that behavior and the consequences of that behavior created distance. In that hotel room in Denver I just felt his presence saying or conveying that he was sorry for some of the difficulties that had been created and that he loved me and he'd done the best he could. I remember crying and releasing something—it was a very good experience. It brought some closure to things that were outstanding, and some of the energy that I had held onto about his dysfunctional behavior dissipated. It was like I was able to forgive and move on. And I was also able to ask for forgiveness because I hadn't been the perfect daughter either.

Jo Anne is an attractive, capable woman in her mid-forties. Her father, too, was an alcoholic.

> My father and I had had virtually no relationship for like twenty years before he died—which was fine with me. He was an alcoholic and a very violent man and separation from him really did nothing but help the quality of my life. My father had gotten polio when he was a child. He was in a wheelchair his whole life and he was very angry. In his time in society, if your legs were crippled, *you* were crippled. Nobody expected much of him—which was a shame because my father had a lot of talents and a lot of intelligence so he was very bitter. Maybe he was just angry with God.
>
> When he got ill and the family realized he was dying—I'm the eldest of five—my mother and the five of us kids went down to the hospital. He had basically kept contact open with everyone else but me and he decided to see everyone else but me before he died, which was okay. I didn't expect the man to have any sudden revelation. I was okay with *my* life and our relationship. So anyway, he passed away. We had a small service and that was that.

I am on the prayer team at my church so I have regular prayer time and prayer practice and one day, months after my father died, I was in prayer without any thought of my father, either that day or for weeks before. All of a sudden I realized that my father was there with me in spirit and it was like a door suddenly had opened. At first I was just shocked. I just sat there in sheer amazement that I was in the middle of this. Then I got to the awareness of what a gift I was being given and I felt incredibly grateful.

His presence stayed with me about three minutes, it was a pretty long length of time, and then suddenly the door closed. During that time I came to know that my father really did love me. It was sudden and unexpected and unplanned-for. It went beyond apology. It was a pureness of love.

Rosemary never felt close to her father. As one of four children, she sought his attention but never quite got it.

His death didn't make a lot of difference to me. He had been sick quite a while, there was sorrow but it was no big deal. Soon after he died, within a day or two, I was writing a letter to a guy out of state, someone I'd never been real close to. I started sensing what at first I thought was this man's affection for me, a lot more than I'd ever sensed before. Suddenly it's as if a voice started yelling at me, "No, not *him. Me!*" And I knew it was my father.

My father was telling me how much he loved me. I sensed this tremendous warmth, it was really, really powerful. I danced all around the living room. I never sensed his touch, he was just there. I remember he was telling me he loved me very much and I swirled around the living room with my dad.

Reconciliation is a recurring theme in after-death contacts. As the first account in the next chapter attests, even the spirit of a dead child who in life seemed hostile may visit to express his love for the living.

8

After the Death of a Child

THE DEATH OF A CHILD evokes a special kind of anguish. This chapter contains stories I've collected from several parents who've sensed contact with their departed child. But sometimes even people who are not blood relatives have ADCs with other people's children who have passed on. The son of Phyllis's friend passed on when he was in his early teens.

> He had a progressive disease, some kind of nerve thing. I didn't know him real well but I had a few moments of contact with the boy at some point or another during his life and it seemed to me that he felt kind of hostilely toward me. So anyway, after the boy passed away I had a dream that he was very, very loving and he was hugging me good-bye. It was a beautiful, beautiful feeling. When I saw the parents, I told them about this dream I'd had and they said that a lot of people had reported to them also having had dreams of him hugging them and telling them good-bye. Sort of like making peace with people and letting them know that everything was okay.

Often sensitives receive messages for someone else. In this case, the psi experiences of people who were *not* related to the lost boy helped his parents to accept his passing.

After the six-year-old son of Maxine's friend died in a grotesque accident, she had a long series of dreams in which he communicated with her. Maxine is a beautiful and sensitive woman who went to a Waldorf school as a child. She grew up taking for granted the reality of other planes of existence.

In 1986, the son of a very close friend of mine was run over accidentally by the boy's father. He was six years old and he was a very fiery sort of a little boy who had a temper. Very angry, very wilful. And he was the third child of four.

Our families were connected in a number of ways. When my husband and I were newly married, we had converted his parents' garage to a little apartment. Then I took care of this boy, Jimmy, in exchange for rent. Well, in 1986 in January, Jimmy's parents separated and this handful of a child went to live with Tom, his father, down the street and his mother, Libby, had the three girls. It was strange, very difficult. By this time, we had moved out of the garage. Then we heard how he had died.

He and his dad were in a truck and they went to a car wash and there was another man with them, a man named Glenn. Jimmy wanted to get out with Glenn. So Glenn and little Jimmy got out and his dad said, "Jim, stay here, I have to go back up the truck into the stall. Don't move. Stay here." So his dad's in the truck driving and Jimmy's standing with the man, Glenn. Tom gets into the truck to move it into the car wash stall and as he's backing up, Jim, as if it was intentionally, he ran behind the truck and the truck ran over him.

Glenn screamed. Tom didn't know what had happened and he was getting out of the truck and Glenn said, "Stop, don't get out of the truck," but by then it was too late. Jimmy was killed instantly. It ran right over his head.

When I heard, I remember not being able to breathe, and feeling as if I had lost my own child. I was in shock. I was 21. He died toward the end of January. Starting the first of February until around November, I had dreams of him virtually every night. Or experiences where I would wake up at 3 in the morning and feel that he was right at the foot of my bed.

The dreams were several. Many, many dreams. And they were all extremely euphoric. Because of them, I felt so relieved. That year they always had him still as a little boy, very happy, but very mature in his countenance. Even though he was a little boy, he was a very wise little boy. And the messages that he would say were, "I'm fine, I'm happy. Don't worry about me. Everything is under control. And tell Libby. Be sure to tell Libby."

There were dreams where he'd be standing in a beautiful field, the classic sort of threshold. I was walking, coming out of a forest and there was a beautiful meadow of little yellow buttercups and bright, rich red poppies. And there he was standing with his very gold, shiny blond hair with nothing on, just waving. Just being. Nothing on and waving—that's how he was—and saying, "I'm happy. I'm okay."

Or I would be at a parade and feeling the sense of excitement and there he would come being hoisted in the air by other children on a canopy thing. And again waving and flowers and just parading and saying, "All is well and I'm great." So these very strong dreams that "I'm okay and tell my mother."

When I had the dreams, I always called up Libby the next morning and said, "Here's the latest." And on many occasions we would have very similar dreams. Dreaming about him, I felt, was normal but the fact that we would have similar experiences in our dreams on the same night, that was very interesting to me.

But the month after he died, I became pregnant. And it was conflicting to be pregnant and to be having these experiences of contact with Jimmy. It was very difficult, I was losing sleep. So finally I put the question out there, I said, "This really has to stop. I can't keep losing sleep like this." I strongly put it out there and it did stop. And I think it sort of waned for Libby. We didn't share as much. It seemed to have a natural completion.

After my daughter was born, I dreamt about him a couple times a year over the next several years. He was still a little boy but there was this wisdom about him that kept maturing and maturing. I felt I was helping him but he could help me too. I'd talk to him. If I was having a situation that I wasn't sure of, I'd say, "Okay, Jim, I need some help here. What's going on?" It's not like he gave me advice in words but through a mood or a feeling, and in the very end he was a full-fledged man. And said "my work is done." It was a real completion. That was the last time that I felt I could call on him for help.

Martin is a Navy veteran who has worked most of his life in the auto repair business and now expresses his substantial artistic abilities by creating beautiful objects out of metal. The father of one child by his first marriage, he and his second wife adopted several children and had one biological son together. Then this son, Perry, died suddenly at the age of 19. About three weeks later, Martin had the only psi experience he could recall ever having.

I went to bed around 10 o'clock. My wife was in bed with me and the dog was in the room. I went to sleep for awhile and woke up around 11 o'clock with a bright light beside my bed. It seemed like something was leaning over me—not a full sized person but smaller. And this light was *bright,* very very bright, like a fluorescent light. It was maybe 20 inches wide and four or five feet high. I wasn't afraid, I was just flat paralyzed really, I could not move. It paused for a moment, sort of wiggled back and forth, then swirled from the room.

I didn't relate this to my wife until noon the next day as we sat weeping in the backyard. I would come home for lunch, we'd cry in the backyard. She told me then that one of our daughters had had a dream that Perry would come back to the room and both of us would see him. I'm the only one who saw him. I was facing this way and she was probably facing the other—and she's a much sounder sleeper than me.

The more I think about it—and believe me I am not one to believe in the supernatural—I think Perry came back to tell me everything was okay, don't worry. Since then my grief has let up a little.

Helen is one of the oldest people I've interviewed but at 78 she looks fifteen years younger. Athletic all her life, she still enjoys walking five miles a day. I interviewed her in the attractive efficiency apartment where she lives by herself. Like Martin, she told me that she'd had wonderful parents with whom she'd enjoyed a happy childhood. Like Martin, she'd had just one paranormal experience—after the death of a beloved child.

Ellen was my youngest. When she was 50, she came down with a mysterious illness. At first they thought it was pneumonia but later they diagnosed it as a rare blood disease. She went so fast! Within five days she was dead.

About two months later, I wasn't thinking about her particularly. I was washing up in my bathroom, getting ready to take my walk, and I started dropping things. Like the toothpaste into the sink, my comb onto the chest of drawers. And that is not me at all, I am not sloppy. I've always been very sure with everything. I was in sports—on the swimming team, pitching on the baseball team—and I move well for my age. It upset me so I looked around and I said over toward the closet, "Ellen, you're playing games with me today. You *never* do that." I never saw her in a playful mood. She had a good sense of humor but it was very esoteric. The moment I said that, a ribbon—

it was not paper but it was stiff enough to be airborne—went from the back of the closet clear out into the living room, going like this. *[Helen wiggled her hand in the air like a fish swimming away from her.]* I never found it, never saw it again. But it was a very pale lavender, her favorite color.

It's not unusual for a psi experience to mirror the real experience of a loved one. In the 1844 Dumas novel, *The Corsican Brothers,* when one twin is shot dead, the other—many miles away—feels such a violent blow on his side that he faints. As Guy Lyon Playfair observed in a recent article, "The idea of a special bond between identical twins that enables them to share sensations at a distance has been widespread for at least 150 years." He went on to cite the case of a 20 year-old woman who, "one day in 1948 . . . felt a massive blow on the left side of her body and a sharp pain. She fell off her chair, cried out to her father, 'Something's happened to Diane', and passed out." Her sister Diane, 70 miles away, had just been in a train crash which left her with two fractured ribs and a concussion. In 1968, Mary had a similar experience—but hers did not involve a twin. It involved her son Bill. At this time he was a young adult.

I was teaching in Thailand in a camp for Cambodian refugees. I was writing on the board and all of a sudden I had like a blow to one side of my head, like someone had hit me or something. It was a sharp, sharp pain and I just sat down and one of my students went and got someone from the office. They took me back to the office. I could barely see, I couldn't even sit up so I lay down on a couch. My head was hurting and I felt terrible.

After two hours, a bus came to take us back home from the camp. My good friend, a Thai man named Preacher, helped me get on, then when we arrived, he helped me get into my room. I didn't feel good at all, he was afraid I'd fall down the steps. I went to sleep, slept very sound. Two or three hours later, Preacher came back and knocked on my door. He woke me up and said I should eat something because I hadn't eaten since breakfast—this was like 2 or 3 in the afternoon. The restaurant was right next door, we went and had soup. We were just sitting in the living room talking when a man and a woman who managed the Save the Children group who were teaching in that refugee camp came to the door. They took me to sit with them at a picnic table outside. That was when they told me, "Your son is dead."

All they knew was that Bill drowned. I wanted to call my parents in Missouri to find out what had happened to him. There weren't many telephones in town so they told me I should probably go into Bangkok and call from there.

I had to go on a Thai bus. I had no idea where to get off and change and I didn't speak the local language that well so they sent a woman that worked in the office along with me. I remember that we rode on top of a truck, on the outside sitting on top of something, and she got me to Bangkok. We took a taxi to the Save the Children office, then I went in and started calling right away from the office.

It was a different time zone, Thailand was twelve hours different. I called my folks and found out that Bill had been in Sacramento, California. He'd gotten a job on Monday. He was gonna start work on Tuesday. So he told the people he was staying with, "I got the job so let's go swimming"—this was in the Sacramento River. I've never seen it but they tell me it's quite a rushing river. He fell off the top of the rocks and he must've hit his head. He was in the water for several minutes. He was still alive when they got him out but he died later, at 11 o'clock at night on Monday in Sacramento and it was Wednesday in Thailand when this happened to me. So it was clearly after he died.

Mary's story sounds a lot like a death coincidence but because the actual times involved were somewhat unclear, I never counted it as one for purposes of my research. What's virtually certain, though, is that belatedly Mary experienced the blow that her son felt when he fell.

A few months before I interviewed Connie, her 35 year-old daughter died unexpectedly of an aneurysm. Connie, who is intensely psychic, has had ADCs of many kinds with her daughter, Irene.

My daughter died last March and I've had quite a lot of communication with her. It's nothing ever really lengthy but like she'll say, "I'm here, mom." Or something will come up and I'll feel a bitter-sweet memory of Irene and she'll say, "Hey, mom, I'm okay. I'm really all right." I'll hear it in her voice and I'll sense her presence. I have contact with her every day in one way or another. I know she's fine, I know she's comfortable. What I really miss is the touch because we were very tactile, we hugged a lot.

Three, four weeks ago I was at a workshop and I was thinking, I really would like to feel her touch—and just at that moment, I felt like someone put their hands on my shoulders behind me. It made the hair on the back of my neck stand straight up. *Ooh,* it really kind of startled me! And I got the telepathic message from her then, "I'm here, mom."

A really interesting thing happened right after she died. You know how you're always grasping for something, like Give me a sign. Well, I live out in the country and I have a lot of hummingbirds. I've lived there for 25 years. I'd never had a personal experience with a hummingbird ever but I was changing the hummingbird feeder, was putting it up, and a hummingbird landed on my finger. I was so mesmerized by it that I stood there for quite a long time and it didn't move. My arm got tired and I went ahead and connected the hummingbird feeder to the ceiling and the hummingbird just jumped off my finger onto the feeder and just watched me. And I just knew that it was some kind of indication from her. Afterwards I felt very calm, very connected.

One of the things that has been really interesting with my daughter is even when I don't ask for any communication, some-times I get it. Like I had to have her cat put to sleep. It was an older cat and the vet didn't feel that it would integrate into another family and I had five young cats and he said that wouldn't work at all. So I really agonized over that and kept trying to think, What would she want? What would she want? I'm really attached to animals so it was really difficult for me to do but I went ahead and as I was driving home, I heard, "Thanks, mom." It was kind of a confirmation that I did the right thing. And I kind of asked her on some of the decisions I made about disposing of her things and I got direction.

I had quite a time at Irene's house when I was trying to take care of things. She had a big three bedroom home that was loaded with stuff. I would put something somewhere and then it wouldn't be there. I had a girlfriend that was helping me. She told me that I was bewitched.

Irene had a really pretty, like a powder box that she really liked—she kept jewelry in it. It had an adorable flowered glass top and that kept getting misplaced. I started feeling she was playing with me. We were extremely close, she's my only child, and she was extremely playful. Then there were all her kitty things. She collected little cat trinkets and statues. There was one that I had bought her that she really liked, a white cat that resembled one of the cats that she loved that had died of old age. That one kept moving around from a little dresser in her bedroom to another little counter in the bathroom where she had stuff. It always stayed in that area but it would go back and forth. It really got to a point where it was kind of amusing and I looked forward to some of those little things. It was a contact.

Connie reported several paranormal incidents which had symbolic significance for her. Like me, she became aware that objects that might have particular meaning were moving from place to place in extraordinary ways. Accounts of similar experiences, reported to me by other interviewees, appear in Chapter 9. Other informants reported experiences which, like Connie's with the hummingbird, involved extraordinary behavior by a living creature. Their stories appear in Chapter 10.

In both of the following cases, mothers lost children in auto accidents. Later they had contact experiences with them. Dorothy is a successful professional in her sixties. Eleven years before I interviewed her, her daughter Amy, a college student, had been killed in a crash in July 1987.

I'm a person of faith and I kept saying to God, most often when I was getting into bed at night, "May I talk to Amy?" And I kept getting no for an answer. Once I asked, "Will I ever be allowed to talk to her?" And the answer I got was, "You may not ask that question." [Laughs] So I kept asking to talk to her and one night in August or September that same year I said a casual, "May I talk to Amy?"—and there she was.

She was magnificent. Her hair just the way I always wanted it to look. Her hair used to be a bone of contention. Now it was lovely, gently curling. And she said, "I'm sorry you're so sad." She told me she was fine. Her presence was calm, gentle, soothing, her anger and tension gone. And I said, "When can I join you?" And she said,

"There's something you have to do." So I said, "Is it this? is it that?" I can't even remember what the five things I asked about were but they were five because they rolled off my fingers that way. She just grinned and left. *[Laughter]* So I've been working very hard since, trying to do whatever it is I'm supposed to do!

Then a little while later, maybe weeks, maybe months, again I was in bed and I said, "I wonder where Amy is, I wonder if she's here." And you know the way the sky looks when it's all gray but you can see the cloud pattern on the bottom, a gray and whitish sort of thing, no big wind? Well, I was within that kind of an atmosphere and Amy had her arm around me as you do when you're saving someone's life and you're trying to head for shore. She was supporting me in that cloudlike substance and it was so good to feel her presence. Nowadays anytime I ask, I am usually granted an awareness of her presence. She's usually here on my left but we haven't said any more words.

Seven years before I interviewed Ut, her daughter died.

She was eleven and a half when we were in a car accident. My memory of it is basically what people filled in because I had severe head injuries. We were hit on her side by a pickup truck going about 55 or 60 miles an hour. She was killed instantly from what I was told. My other children were in the back seat. She had asked to sit in the front that morning. . . .

About a month or so after she died, the grief was overwhelming. One night after everyone else had gone to bed I was sitting at the kitchen table alone just crying. I decided I couldn't go on. I can't say I was actually contemplating suicide because I wasn't saying *how* I was gonna end it but the thought kept going through my mind that it was too much pain, I couldn't go on. And I got this shudder, a chill.

I remembered hearing that when you get little ones like that, somebody just walked across your grave and I just blew it off but a few minutes later it happened again and it happened so strongly that it literally pushed me into the kitchen table. I looked up and for some reason I knew and I said, "Jenny?" I knew that she had been there, that she had touched me. And the next morning when I woke up, I had more strength and energy than I had had since it happened. And I knew that she had reached out and gave me some of her strength, letting me know I had to go on. To this day there's times when things get difficult and I'll get that same shudder through me and I know it's her. I just look up and say, "I love you."

There've been other things. That first year I went to work for a company doing some telemarketing and it turned out that these people had a son who died of muscular dystrophy when he was 21, about a year before Jenny did. So it was very good to get to work with somebody that understood what I was going through. But what was amazing was there was times that—and I kind of freaked out at first—the copy machine was upstairs in another room and it would just go on all by itself when *nobody* was there. I looked at my boss and said, "Judy?" and she goes, "Oh, yeah, that's Eddie, he's playing a trick." Her son. She'd noticed that these things happened quite often. Then we decided, oh probably it's *both* of the kids having fun with us. You'd be downstairs and all of a sudden this copy machine would start up. There was no paper in it, it wasn't making a copy of anything, it was just going. It only happened when we were in the office alone. Either me by myself or her by herself or the two of us together. That's why we would look at each other and say the kids are playing jokes on us. I think it's kinda neat. They make their presence known in little ways.

9

Lights That Blink a Message

ELECTRICALLY OPERATED DEVICES like that copying machine seem tailor-made to convey messages from spirits. The dead often communicate with the living by systematically disturbing electromagnetic fields—most commonly by signaling with our ever-present electric lights. This book's first chapter described how, when my husband Paul started losing his vision, he bought himself a particularly powerful floor lamp by which he could still read. Soon after Paul died, my son and I saw his lamp turn itself on and flash in what seemed to be a meaningful fashion. It appeared to have difficulty flashing unless we were fairly close to it. In 1916 Sir Oliver Lodge, a distinguished British physicist and a fellow of the Royal Society, wrote about a related phenomenon.

By that time, Lodge had been a devoted student of the paranormal for many years. In 1909, he authored a book in which he expressed his belief that the human personality could survive death. In the spirit world after death, he asserted, "memory, culture, education, habits, character and affection . . . and to a certain extent tastes and interests . . . are retained [while for the most part] worldly possessions, bodily pain and disabilities . . . fall away." He dedicated this work to "the founders of the Society for Psychical Research: the truest and most patient workers in an unpopular region of science that I have ever known."

Then in 1915, Lodge's youngest child, Raymond, was killed in World War I. Now Sir Oliver, like many another British parent who lost a loved one in that bloody conflict, started visiting mediums—including some of the most gifted ones of his era—in an effort to contact his son. More than once, he succeeded. In his 1916 book, *Raymond,* he tells of many kinds of seances—often called "sittings"—in which he received communications. Most interesting with regard to electromagnetic fields was one which Lodge referred to as a "table sitting." Here communication came via movements of a small table, 18 inches square, at which Lodge and his wife were seated along with the medium and one other person. It was agreed that in response to the sitters' questions, the table would tilt three times for "yes" and once for "no." For more complex messages, the medium recited the alphabet and the spirit communicator tilted the table at each one. When a letter was called and the table did *not* tilt, that letter was written down as part of the message. A fifth sitter, seated at another table, served as recorder.

Lodge was a man of science. His son, who was 26 when he died, had been trained as a mechanical and electrical engineer. Midway in the seance, Sir Oliver asked his son, "Can you explain how you do this? I mean, how you work the table?" Raymond's answer came back, laboriously spelled letter by letter, YOU ALL SUPPLY MAGNETISM GATHERED IN MEDIUM AND THAT GOES INTO TABLE AND WE MANIPULATE. Just as my son and I had guessed when Paul's lamp first flashed in our presence, *we* ourselves were contributing factors to its flashing—but only as unwitting sources for some kind of magnetic energy. Probably lots of spirit manifestations involve just such monkeying with magnetic fields. Though science has yet to trace the process, step by step, there's ample evidence that this process exists.

A third of my interviewees reported paranormal experiences that involved electric lights or other electrically operated devices. In earlier chapters we've heard from four of them about lights that behaved in extraordinary fashion.

Sara and Spring, half-sisters who'd lost their brother John, were both at John's mother's house when the kitchen light which had been turned up as high as it ordinarily went, suddenly got much brighter. Though Sara didn't directly witness that brightening light, at the very same time she received telepathic directions which helped her to at last find a missing video. Taken together, the two events snared the attention of everyone present. Also reported in Chapter 3 was Anna's story of finding hidden chocolate at the home of her recently deceased aunt, thanks to a telepathic message from her aunt's spirit which first announced its presence to Anna by blinking lights. Then in Chapter 4, we heard from Denise about her travails with her late ex-husband's spirit. Three times when she was alone in bed with her current husband, the two of them were awakened by their bedroom light turning on.

Linda told me a story about shenanigans with lights—and microphones—that engaged the attention of hundreds of people. I interviewed her together with her husband, Steven. He also had witnessed this event and he backed up Linda's account as she gave it to me.

I had a very dear friend named Sherry Wong. I met her soon after she was diagnosed with cancer but she wasn't the sort that would take it lying down. For five years she battled it and I got to know her very well. She was the kind of person who took the best from every religion. She would go to the Mormon Church and the Catholic Church—her husband was Catholic—and she'd go to the Seventh Day Adventists. She just took the best from everybody, put it all together and had her own little form of religion. She had many many friends and her motto was When the Lord gives you lemons, make lemonade.

We grew very close, really like sisters. Almost to the point where my family suffered because every time I stopped by to see her, Sherry wouldn't let me go. About a month before she passed away she said to me, "Linda, I don't know how I'm gonna do it yet, but I know you're all gonna be worried about me when I'm gone. Somehow I'm gonna let you know I'm okay."

The Sunday after she died we had a big service, celebration service, Sunday night service at St. Jude's. The place was packed and they're getting ready for the service to begin—and suddenly the lights go out. And all the power, all the microphones, nothing's working in the sanctuary. People are running around. There's no reasonable reason why anything is not working. The lights are on everywhere else around the church.

Well, there were probably five of us who were the closest to Sherry and we all looked at each other. It was like we all realized at the same time that this was Sherry's way. Only someone like that could intervene in the system to make this happen. There's nothing like a blackout to get everybody's attention. So we all said at the same time, "Sherry's okay." Then just as suddenly as the lights had gone out, they came back on again. So the service proceeded. The blackout and all that hullabaloo was just like a little fanfare—but that's the way she was. Sherry was very dramatic.

Three years before I interviewed Joan, her father died. She traveled two thousand miles to attend his funeral. That night, while she was staying in his home, she had a very private experience of his presence that affected her deeply.

I was sitting in his chair at about four in the morning. Just sort of grieving and mourning and not able to sleep. My husband was asleep in the other room, my mother was upstairs. And the porch light just went on. I wasn't scared, I didn't jump up from my chair as you would normally react. I just had the sense that it was okay. I just *knew* that it was *him* for some reason. That was really just one of the signs that he was there with me at that point. It didn't stay on long—maybe three, four minutes, something like that. It didn't flash, it just stayed on. It gave me a calm sort of peaceful feeling.

So I talked to my mom the next day. I knew my parents' home so well. I knew they would never put one of those motion things outside but still I checked with her. I said, "Did Dad ever install one of those motion lights?" And of course, just like I figured, she told me no.

Michael wrote me from a village in Britain about a helpful experience he had with lights a few months after his wife passed on.

One evening I decided to go and do some business at a local town the following day, making an early start by getting up at 7:30. However I stayed up late watching a football match, and I would have overslept the next day except I was awakened by a bright light shining in my eyes. It was the bedside lamp on my wife's side of the bed. This lamp had not been on since my wife's death, to the best of my recollection. It was operated by two switches, one on the wall and one on the lamp. I got up immediately, walked round the bed and switched the lamp off, and noticed at the same time that it was 7:30.

Can one style of communicating after death run in a family? Pat told me a series of stories that suggest this can happen. After her father-in-law died, her husband, Richard—an electrical engineer—sensed that his father was signaling to him through street lights that blinked as he approached.

Around eighteen months after his father died, Richard said to me, "I don't know what he's trying to say but I can be driving at night somewhere and a street light'll blink and I think of Dad." He wanted to know what I thought and I said, "Well, I don't know, but if you get a warm feeling with it, it's certainly not anything to worry about." And he says, "I kinda worry about my sanity!" And I said, "You're still as sane as you've ever been, don't worry about that!"

So then a year and a half later, my husband died. *[When he died, after a long battle with cancer, they had been married for 32 years.]* My oldest son was working extra hours for an accounting firm and he never got home before dark. And he said sometimes he'd be driving home and have as many as eight of the street lights blink on the way, and he says to me, "That's too many, that's statistically impossible." So we went over what his father thought about his grandfather trying to communicate with him and I told him, "Your dad got some comfort out of it and I hope you'll look at it that way, too." So all this leads up to what happened to me. This happened to me soon after my husband's passing.

Richard wanted to die at home. I live in a very large house with no bedrooms on the entry level. He passed away in the dining room because that was the only room we could turn into something comfortable for him. A few days after he died, it was twilight and I thought I'd do a little meditation. Some background music would be nice. And that was in the room my husband passed away in. I went over to the stack and I couldn't see well enough to pick out a CD. So I turned the light on and the most amazing thing happened! It was like blue light was jumping all the way around the chandelier. It has five or six small bulbs shaped like candle flames? Normally anything electric that goes bonkers just scares me to death because I don't understand electricity. *[Laughs]* But anyway I'm there and I watch this. It was flashing around from bulb to bulb! And I'm thinking, "How can this be?"

So I quickly turned it off because I didn't know what else to do and then I thought, you know, that was really pretty. It was beautiful, not threatening. So I turned it back on and nothing happened. It was like the whole thing was blown. So I went out in the garage and checked the circuit. No, the circuit wasn't blown. So I went ahead and put the music on and sat in my chair and I kept thinking and thinking. And I thought, my husband was an electrical engineer and this is the room he died in. And he told me, "If there's a way, I'll communicate with you."

Barbara has had many experiences with wildly behaving lights. She believes the communicator is her mother and she's understandably proud of her.

Barbara's mother—also named Barbara—came from a wealthy family descended from the Revolutionary War patriot, Samuel Adams. As a young adult she was dogged by alcoholism. Then she joined Alcoholics Anonymous. She stayed sober for the last thirty years of her life and set out to help needy women with substance abuse problems. With a rabbi, a priest and a lawyer she helped found the first alcoholic women's halfway house in Orange County, California and, according to her daughter, she was the first woman in the country to take the AA program into women's prisons.

The younger Barbara is highly sensitive. An astrologer and counselor, she has participated in many workshops on the paranormal. One of them figures in what she told me about the impact of her mother's spirit on lights.

Something that Mother has done has affected lots of people. When something was going to happen in the family, she would start blinking the lights. It would usually be no more than a week before. One I remember that was really pretty dramatic was when our youngest daughter was in Saudi Arabia with our son-in-law. They were working for Lockheed, next door to Iran. And the Saudis closed the whole country down for three weeks when somebody went in there and shot up the mosque at Mecca.

Well, at the time my husband had just installed brand new fluorescent lights overhead in our kitchen. Being an engineer, he freaked because they started blinking. With Mother there are different kinds of blinks. There are frantic blinks and then there are the soft, slow blink ... blink ... blink. This was the frantic blink. It went on for one whole evening from, say, 7:00 until we went to bed around 10:30. Every time I would walk into the kitchen and turn on the lights, they'd do this. My husband was so disgusted with the whole thing that he took all the tubes down and had 'em checked and they were all fine. *[chuckling]* That was what made him a believer. Now when lights blink, he'll just say, "Hi, Barbara."

I was living in Tucson, Arizona when this was happening. Our oldest daughter was attending the university there and had her own apartment. That same evening we compared notes. At precisely the same time my lights started blinking, the lights in the whole library at the university started blinking! Well, quite a few people from Saudi were students there so there were a lot of people that were gonna be affected. But this thing, it's like exponential. It gets big.

Our daughter in Saudi Arabia had her own craziness to deal with. They were ten hours ahead of us so when it was evening for us, for her it was early in the morning the next day. When they woke up they were in their house for about an hour and a half while they were getting ready to go to work and the lights did not stop blinking that whole time. But we didn't find this out until quite a while later. The Saudis closed the country down and for three weeks we could not be in touch.

But here's the topper. I was telling this story in 1983 or '84, at a week-long super-seminar in this giant auditorium. So what do you think Mother did? She dimmed all the lights in the auditorium and blinked them. She really freaked the folks. I mean, there were like 450 people there. And what I heard was, "Ohhhh." *[laughs]* But she was just saying, "Hi there." And then when I was done talking about her, it was like she took a bow. Blink, blink. So what I said into the mike was, "Showoff!"

In Chapters 3 and 4 we heard from Laura, whose husband, Dave, died by his own hand of carbon monoxide poisoning. Then—after much hesitation about moving on to loving judgment from a smoggy netherworld—he started communicating with her and her daughter in a warm, supportive fashion. While Dave was still alive, he urged their mutual friend Steve to take care of Laura if anything happened to him. When, after her husband's death, the relationship between Steve and Laura blossomed, much of Dave's support for this development came via a light.

When he died, we just had a carport. Since then I've enclosed it and put a garage door on it. The electrical wiring was redone. We used to have a fluorescent light we always left on. The contractor took that away and put a different light in. It's a fluorescent with a switch, there's only one switch to it. Believe me, I've gone through my whole house trying to figure out if there's any other switches I could be inadvertently fiddling with.

At first I just kind of noticed that the light was on. I'd go back and turn it off and think, "That's weird, I know I'm not turning it on." I started making a conscientious effort to make sure the light was always off when I wasn't around and the door was locked. I'm the only one with a key to get into the garage.

So then I started seeing a very clear pattern. It only turns on when I've been with Steve. Whether we've gone for dinner or I've spent the night with him or we've had some kind of intimate talk—whatever it is, it's only that time. It never turns on when I've just gone off to the grocery store, for example. It's just the strangest thing.

One night Steve and I were going out to dinner with another couple and Steve's ex-wife confronted us. She just appeared out of nowhere. It was very uncomfortable, an awful situation. We had just been at the house and driven away from there, closed the garage, the whole bit. So we knew the light was off. We had this awful confrontational experience with his ex-wife, then we drive home and the garage door opens up and, what do you know, the light's on. And it's just, *omigod*.

Sometimes I wonder, maybe I should just stop seeing Steve, just get away from here. And every single time I've thought that, I drive home and that light's on. Steve has seen it and my daughter has seen it when she's ridden with me. I picked her up one time and came back home with her after having spent the night out at the lake with Steve. It's like Dave is telling me that what I'm doing with Steve is okay.

Charlie is a college professor who in the past few years has sensed contact with both of his parents and with his grandfather. Stories of some of his ADCs are in Chapters 3 and 4. Not long before I interviewed him, he had a light experience that seemed to him like a gift from his mother and father.

> In my office I have what I call my pop culture museum. It's a batch of little artifacts, and over it I have a whole string of pepper lights. You know what I mean? Christmas lights that look like a string of green chili peppers.
>
> Now the day before my birthday, I had been working around with this little display of mine. And I know for definite sure that I did *not* have the lights plugged into the wall. I would have known. It would have been impossible for me not to see that. Anyhow, I never leave stuff like that plugged in because I'm overly cautious about electrical appliances and stuff that might cause fires. And you have to crawl behind the couch to plug in first the lava lamp—there's a lava lamp up there—and also these pepper lights.
>
> Now the next morning, which was my birthday, they're lit up. You know how it is when people sense a subjective meaning? An intuitive connection? Well, I just knew my parents had done that to say, "Happy Birthday." It was like the candles on the cake.
>
> Meanwhile the skeptical part of my mind was trying to figure out, "What could this be?" But who's going to come in my office and plug those in? The only person who would even have a key and come in would be the person that comes in to empty the wastebasket. And they're not going to fool around with plugging my lights in, for Pete's sake! I mean, it's a hassle even to get to it. And there's no motivation whatsoever, even though it's possible. Plus the date it happened was such a super coincidence. So I just felt real tickled at that. It meant a lot to me to have my parents say, "Happy Birthday."

Lights catch our eyes, to say the least. They grab our attention. But as the next chapter shows, paranormal events that involve other electrical devices can have plenty of impact too.

10

Misbehaving Radios, Telephones—and More

A<small>NY HONEST RESEARCH STUDY</small> has an element of randomness to it. Unless you're dealing with thousands of cases, you can be pretty sure that your data will *not* present a perfectly balanced picture of the real world. Some aspects will be overestimated, others will be underestimated. For instance, if you toss a coin fifty times, it's unlikely that you will get heads—or tails—exactly twenty-five times, though probably the tallies for your two categories will be more or less equal. It's even more unlikely that your coin will fall first heads, then tails, then heads, then tails throughout your study. In fact, the chance of this happening in a run of fifty consecutive coin tosses is less than one in a *quadrillion* (1,000,000,000,000,000). Of course it's staggeringly hard even to conceive of such a number since a quadrillion is *a thousand thousand billion.*

Twenty-one people in my study reported paranormal experiences that involved electrical gadgets aside from lights. Not surprisingly, telephones and radios were mentioned most often. But I was startled—though not disturbed—to find that for two of them the gadget involved was an electronic keyboard. Here is what Summer, the dance teacher and dance ethnologist quoted earlier, told me about hers.

> I play piano and I had a funky old electric piano that definitely had a ghost in it. It was really strange. It would turn on a different

124

voice just me wanting it to happen. It would change before I pressed the button to change it. It was almost as if I could control it telepathically—except that sometimes I wasn't totally in control. I had a real love-hate relationship with it because it didn't always do what I wanted it to. It had its own head. Amazing. I've had similar experiences with my cars. I have old cars and I hang onto my cars and have a relationship with them. Name 'em and everything. . . .

I had that keyboard for years. Hardly anybody else used it, it was finicky. What I'm saying is that there was some kind of spirit connection between it and myself which makes me believe what the mystics say about, you know, we're all one. I have many musician friends and composers who say they were given a song by God or the spirit and often historically composers have said things like that. Music and dance are very connected to spirit.

Mary-Minn told me this similar story.

I used to play the piano really seriously. I never got very good at it but I practiced hours and hours a day. Then I got a bad back injury and couldn't play the piano but around that time a fellow named Charles, a friend of my husband's, was working on a keyboard he'd invented. It was a way of interfacing a keyboard with a computer. Charles and a programmer were building a music composition program that they hoped they'd be able to sell. I was beta testing it. Could a beginner play with this? Well, I was a beginner and yes, a beginner could. He was training me on it and I was having fun playing on his keyboard. Not composing, just improvising.

He had it up in a loft, on a raised platform. One day I was up there with Charles, the inventor, who was a fine musician. I hadn't been playing but the sound system was on and suddenly a short composition came out. It was not something Charles could have done. It was definitely not good enough to be his composition and it wasn't his style but it was very similar to mine—only it was better than stuff I played. It didn't have all that technical clumsiness I had because I really was a beginner. It was the way I *wanted* to play, fettered only by my imagination, not by my bad coordination and my lousy keyboard skills.

This piece lasted about a minute and Charles and I looked at each other. We figured maybe, just maybe, someone else had been playing around and had stored it in the computer but when we tried to retrieve it, we couldn't. It wasn't there. Another weird thing about it, I held on to the experience and Charles was amazed by it for about half an hour but then he forgot all about it. I mean, he didn't even remember it the next day.

Mary-Minn's husband is a brilliant theoretical physicist. He was present while she told me this story and confirmed it for me. Like many physicists, he is an open-minded man confident of his abilities to assess the basic verities of our world, no matter how far his conclusions may stray from the accepted "wisdom" of the day.

Britain's Society for Psychical Research, matrix for some of the world's most significant studies of the paranormal, has counted among its numbers many shining lights in the natural sciences since its founding over a century ago. In fact, it was a physics professor interested in Spiritualist phenomena, William Barrett, who first convinced an elite circle of Fellows at Trinity College, Cambridge University, that the society should be established.

Sir Oliver Lodge, who was knighted for his work as a physicist, served several terms as president of the SPR. (Lodge helped lay the foundation for wireless telegraphy and ultimately for radio.) Similarly, during the early part of the twentieth century a distinguished French astronomer, Camille Flammarion, authored a series of books on paranormal phenomena. Encouraged by his interest in the subject, over the course of half a century, thousands of people from around the world wrote him about their uncanny experiences—which often involved contact with the dead. His three volume study, *Death and Its Mystery*, comprised extensive quotes from hundreds of their letters, many of them accompanied by confirming letters from other witnesses to the events involved. In its concluding chapter, he observed:

> The object of this work has been attained. . . . The occurrences cited, the truth of which has been duly established, prove that there is no death. . . . "Death is the portal of life." The body is but an organic garment of the spirit; it dies, it changes, it disintegrates: the spirit remains. . . . The universe is a dynamism. An intelligent force rules all. The soul cannot be destroyed.

Thomas Henry Huxley, founding genius of a near dynasty of literary and scientific geniuses, was a fearlessly controversial biologist of the latter nineteenth century. A supporter of Darwin's theories of evolution, he inflamed the anger of both scientists and clergy when he argued that anthropoid apes are humankind's closest relatives—a finding which contemporary DNA studies now prove beyond question. How, according to Huxley, should a scientist proceed? "Sit down before fact like a little child," he said, "and be prepared to give up every preconceived notion, follow humbly wherever and to whatever abysses Nature leads you or you shall learn nothing." Unfortunately, the world is full of timid, conformist types who dare not do the same.

Only too believable in Mary-Minn's account is that detail about her friend Charles and his inability to remember what had happened just the day before. Knee-jerk disbelievers are blinded by their prejudices. Imprisoned by their fixed beliefs, they dare not acknowledge what their senses attest is real.

Most of us have contact with telephones virtually every day so it was hardly surprising that several of my interviewees reported having had paranormal experiences that involved them. More than one mentioned that, soon after the death of a loved one, he or she had received a series of hang-up calls. The phone would ring normally so they would pick up, but then nobody would respond at the other end. Did this mean that some spirit presence was trying to get through? Or was some acquaintance just at a loss for words? Or did some real live person at the other end just want to hear the answerer's voice? For the most part, my informants—a level-headed crew—did not leap to the conclusion that such truncated calls were true after-death contacts. The most strongly documented story of a telephone ADC came from Tom, the man whose telepathic experiences after his wife died in an accident are reported at the start of Chapter 3. This is what happened about three weeks after his second wife, Norma, died.

> On the 20th of June, we're in Oregon except that her son stayed in our house up in Washington because he had a job nearby. At 5:50

in the afternoon, the phone rang in Oregon at her girlfriend Denise's house—and Denise had been saying, "I wish Norma would talk to me. I really need her to talk to me." Well, her phone rang. Her granddaughter answered the phone but pretty soon she hung up. So Denise came out and said, "Who was that on the phone?" "There was nobody there," her granddaughter said, "I just heard a woman's sigh, then there was nothing." So Denise said, "Well, let's look at the caller ID and see where this call came from."

Turned out the call came from my home in Washington. She thought that was strange but she knew Norma's son was there and she thought maybe he called and wanted something so she dialed back. It rings in Washington and he answers the phone and she says, "What did you want?" He says, "I didn't want nothing. What are you talking about?" She says, "Well, there was a call from your house and we wanted to know what you wanted." He says, "I don't even know your number and there's been nobody on this phone. Don't play games with me. Are you trying to scare me?" Denise says, "No, but there was a phone call at 5:50."

So Denise told me all this and I said, "When I get my final bill from the telephone company, I'll check that." Sure enough, at 5:50 in the afternoon there was a phone call made from our old place in Washington to Denise's house in Oregon. I got charged 15 cents which I think is the minimum charge.

When I interviewed Tom, just two months after his wife's death, it seemed clear that Norma was a particularly determined communicator from the other side. Electrical appliances provided some of her favorite routes for contact.

Her daughter's microwave went on the blink. Her brother's an electrician, he checked it over, there was nothing wrong with it, it fired back up. Her refrigerator went on the blink, there was nothing wrong with the refrigerator, it started back up. There was nothing he could find. Her daughter was reading this book, *Talking to Heaven*. One of the things it says that happens, your electrical things go bananas.

Norma had an answering machine, her voice was on the greeting. I wanted to keep her voice on that tape so I took it off the machine and put it away. I bought two new tapes, exactly the same, but that thing has not worked right since then. That answering machine will *not work* without her tape. The new tapes sound all garbled. So I told Norma, "I bought a new answering machine. I'm gonna retire yours and I'll put your tape back in there and years from now we'll plug it back in and listen to you."

Last night I was trying to call a woman and *[chuckles]* every time I tried to call, that phone would hang up. All of a sudden I'd get a dial tone and there was no reason for this to happen. So obviously Norma doesn't want me to talk to this woman!

Maria had a more subtle experience with a telephone after a favorite relative died.

This happened to me and my mother. My uncle Ray died and at that time I didn't have a phone. She managed to get in touch with me through a sheriff in Detroit of all things. I was living in Detroit then and she was living in Houston, so I called her on a pay phone. My uncle Ray was her brother, she told me what had happened to him. As we were talking we kept getting not quite disconnected. We kept having to say, "Hello, hello," and "Are you still there?" And I thought, even at that time when I didn't have any notions about any afterlife, I thought that was something like he would do as a joke. He would get some fun out of it.

He was kind of a tease. He liked to do things to amuse people. He was a favorite uncle of ours, particularly when we were little. So it sort of tickled me actually—although I did want to stay connected on the phone, I didn't really want to be cut off. But my first reaction was kind of smiling. It was like something he would do.

After Elsie's mother died, curious things started happening to her telephone that suggested that her mom was getting back at Elsie's errant ex-husband.

I didn't have anything to wear to my mother's funeral so I went shopping in the morning. Now I split with my first husband after 25 years in a very painful divorce. My husband had had a long affair with his graduate assistant and my mother never forgave him. When I came home from the shopping trip, my present husband said, "Oh, Jack called. He wants to know when the memorial service is. I told him when it was but I couldn't give him the exact time." I said, "Oh dear, I'd better phone him." Picked up the phone, the line was totally dead.

We went through 24 hours of checking with the neighbors, nobody else had a problem. I was sure someone had cut the telephone line someplace. Nothing wrong. I reported it to the phone company. They were sending a crew out, couldn't get there for three days. With all the arrangements we were making for the memorial service, it was *very* inconvenient. But it did occur to me that my mother would have *absolutely* cut that line the minute he called.

By around midnight that night I picked up the phone and it was making crackly noises and the next morning it was working. That morning I used the telephone several times but I never did call my ex back. Then when I was preparing salads to take up for the memorial service, the telephone rang and I picked it up and it was dead except for these same crackly noises that I heard. And I said, "Okay, I got it," hung up the phone. And that's all the trouble we had.

Marti reported a series of experiences with her late husband's spirit that involved an *imaginary* phone. They recalled his sense of humor to her but he also seemed to be reaching her a helping hand.

In the last house I lived in, there was a garage that I used as an office and I slept in a loft above the garage. There weren't any phones in that part of the house but I remember being up in the loft once and hearing the phone—like it was ringing down in the kitchen. I went down and picked up the phone and the phone wasn't ringing. I told a friend that Wayne had installed some sort of intergalactic phone line.

Generally when I hear a phone when there isn't a phone ringing, he does in fact have something to tell me. I'm very strong-willed and strong-minded. He's one of the few people that I've ever known that I trusted, that when he had some kind of input to give me, I just listened. That's still true. Usually I sit and go into some kind of meditative trance, just try to be open to whatever comes. The last time I can remember, it was about a man I was going out with. Wayne believed with some reason that I had certain blind spots and naivete about men and he had this marvelous way of being able to give me input without me getting my hackles up. It almost felt like he was a good older brother. So the last time I can remember specifically the phone call thing it was about my relationship with a guy that I was seeing at the time.

I asked Marti, "When you go into a meditative state and you're listening for advice, how long are the messages you receive?" Her answer was, "Short—ten words or less. To the point. They catch my attention." This recalls numerous other accounts reported in this book. Again and again, informants said they'd received a few pithy words of wisdom that nonetheless had immense impact for them. Similarly, the typical sense of presence experience, however moving, seems to last just three or four minutes.

I myself have never received verbal messages from a departed spirit; generally I've had to puzzle out the meanings of physical clues from my beloved punster spirit, Paul. But on several occasions in recent years I've received terse, even slangy directives in response to prayers for guidance.

Yes, I do pray. I pray a lot. Though at the time of my late husband's death in 1983 I was a confirmed agnostic, my repeated experiences of spirit contact thereafter led me to different, greener pastures and, in time, to a new faith. The first time I attended the Quaker meeting where I am now a member, I was deeply troubled. A longtime close associate who had often treated me unkindly, hurtfully, had fumbled herself into a life threatening situation. Time and again for weeks, against all my ethical standards, I found myself wishing her dead—even as I recognized that such feelings were unacceptable. Sitting with a roomful of others in silent meditation, I laid my problem in the hands of the Great Spirit. Softly but persistently, the answer came to me, repeating again and again in my head, "Pray that she will treat you better."

Just seven words—but they solved my problem. Why, I wondered, had I never thought of that before? Perhaps because never before had I believed in the power of prayer. That Sunday morning, I started praying that this longtime thorn in my side would survive—and would treat me more lovingly in the future. Wonder of wonders, she did! Basking in the sunshine of her transformation, I soon became a Quaker by convincement.

Marti, quoted above, has a son named Grant. In Chapter 5, I cited a sense of presence experience he had with his father's spirit while he was a teenager on a hiking trip. Years later, on the night before his wedding to Elaine, Grant sensed that he was contacted via a radio. Then just before the wedding ceremony, once again he sensed his father's presence.

> We woke up in the middle of the night with our radio on. It must've been between two and three in the morning and we hadn't set the alarm but there was a voice on the radio and I believe it was my dad. Elaine remembers that I told her it sounded like my dad. That's the only time I've actually heard him say anything since he died. Elaine woke up too. We both heard directions, directions in a navigational sense. It was like a procedure being narrated. I used to keep a journal. I wish I'd kept better track of it.
>
> Then that day we were getting ready for the wedding. We were getting married at the arboretum. I'd gone back home to get dressed and was driving our Volvo out to the arboretum. I don't know what got me thinking about my dad but I felt that he was sitting in the car with me. Once again he didn't really say anything to me but I felt he was there in the passenger seat. It was remarkable. I remember trying to think of something to ask or just to key in. What do I need to ask you? What do I need to do here? I don't feel I got a specific response. I feel like I was acknowledged. I knew that he was there for me.

Favorite songs often figure in radio ADCs. For instance, a woman in Roberta Conant's study of Massachusetts widows described a particularly depressing day she'd spent searching from store to store for hard to match replacement parts for the bathroom of a rental apartment. This was a job her late husband would have done. Just when her morale had sunk to its lowest ebb, her car radio played one of their favorite songs. She dared it to play their other favorite—and that's what came on next. For her, this was an unmistakable sign of her husband's encouragement.

One of the most intricate stories I collected came to me from Jo, a confident, sometimes jovial woman, the mother of six and a retired school librarian with a master's degree and many additional graduate credits. Weirdly behaving radios—and other material objects—played important roles in finally resolving a heart-wrenching family problem.

I was starting a new job at an elementary school and I had a workshop before school. A number of funny things started happening in my environment. I didn't pay particular attention to them until one day I came home and books from the top of my book shelf had mysteriously fallen down. Dante's *Inferno* was open on the couch. I thought of all these other funny things I'd been noticing so I called my son who had been in the house that day. He said, "Mom, I was right there when it happened. Those books jumped off the shelf, you must have a poltergeist." The two of us laughed and laughed over it.

Later I was telling this story to a friend. She told me, "Jo, you should try something like a ouija board." Well, it happened that in my children's games that I'd been storing, we did have a ouija board so I said, "All right, if you'll do it with me, I'll try it." We got what I thought was a lot of gibberish. After she left, I looked again at what I'd written down and what popped out at me was the numeral "4" and the first initial and last name of my sister-in-law.

Now my sister-in-law Marilyn had been grieving mightily for seven years since her 21 year-old daughter died after giving birth to a baby. We'd lost contact with that baby, the father was not somebody we could deal with. This was a great worry, what had happened to that child? The reason I was paying attention to these funny things was that years ago I had read a book by Bishop Pike, *The Other Side*. After his son died, lots of strange things had happened to him too and he was a really brilliant man. He'd been a top-notch lawyer before he became a bishop [in the Episcopal Church.]

Well as I said, because I was doing this workshop, I had to get up very early. I set my radio alarm clock and in the middle of the night, my radio alarm turned on. I thought, my gosh, how did I foul up on that? Turned on the light. Tried to turn off the radio and it couldn't be turned off, simply couldn't be turned off. I finally had to unplug it from the wall and hope I woke up on time. I thought a lot about this. Seemed to me like somehow my niece was trying to get in touch with me about this child.

Now my sister-in-law, my mother-in-law, that whole family were arch skeptics, very down to earth people. I worried about approaching them with something so unscientific as this. But on Saturday I phoned my mother-in-law and said, "Look, these funny things are happening to me. I think I need to tell Marilyn." And she said, "Oh please don't. Marilyn has been through so much. I wouldn't like you to bring something like that up." Marilyn was my sister-in-law whose daughter had died.

The minute I hung up the phone, the radio turned on and I couldn't turn it off without unplugging it. I didn't pay attention to what it was playing but it was music. So I said, "Okay, that's it." I arranged to have my sister-in-law meet me for breakfast. I told her and she did not hoot at me as I'd expected her to. She said, "Let's go back to your house and try that ouija board."

So we did and the planchette started moving at such speed that I took my hands off. I didn't want to be accused of moving it. I simply recorded. It was a rather brief message from my niece to her mother and the essence of it was, "I'm okay, I want you to be happy. I want *you* to get along with your life." At one point Marilyn stopped and took her hands off the planchette. We both laughed because Marilyn said, "I can see where this sentence is going." Then she put her hand back on the planchette and it proceeded to spell out that message without interruption even though we had both gotten it and we both hooted because this was totally, "Don't interrupt, mother!"

This profoundly affected Marilyn. She went back to school and got another master's in religious education. She began to explore these things. Years after the event that caused my sister-in-law to change her way of thinking, her mother died. My mother-in-law had remained a skeptic. The day after the memorial service, I got a phone call from my sister-in-law and she said, "I want you to sit down for this. I got a phone call a few minutes ago from a woman who said, "I am the adoptive mother of this child..."—that everyone was looking for, that everyone was so concerned about. "And she said, 'This is crazy that I'm making this phone call. My husband and I promised that when our daughter was 19 we would give her this information but not before. But for the last few days I have just been *weighted* with a feeling that I have to call you.'" And Marilyn responded with, "Oh, I think I understand why." [Chuckling]

So they arranged to meet for lunch. After this meeting, my sister-in-law called me. She said, "You won't believe it. I told her as we started lunch that when my mother died, if there was one thing she would try to bring about, it would be to put us in touch with each other." And the woman said, "I know what you mean. I never knew what I thought about that until *my* mother died a few years ago and that night all of a sudden the radio turned on all by itself and it was playing her favorite song."

Now that family is back together again and the grandparents are back in contact with that child. It was strange how the woman knew how to contact Marilyn. Marilyn had gone to a convention a hundred miles from where she lived. The adoptive mother of this child was involved in setting it up. Someone came up to her and said, "Will you please staff Registration for me while I go to the bathroom?" So she just sat down. The first person to come along was my sister-in-law and the adoptive mother recognized her name from the adoption papers and saved her address. That's how she knew how to get in touch with her.

You know that expression: There are just a dozen people in the world—the rest is done with mirrors.

11

Symbolic Events

AGAIN AND AGAIN WE SEE THE SAME PATTERN. The dead reach out to the living. They try to help them, guide them, comfort them with evidence of their affection. If one route doesn't work, they try another. Sometimes they have to send their message through a more perceptive person. In this chapter we will look at events— physical and psychic—that conveyed deep meanings to the people who received them.

Elise is a true sensitive; at times she has even served as a medium. When her first marriage was in difficulty, her husband's late grandfather used her as a conduit for a warning to his grandson.

My ex-husband, Jimmy, and I pulled into a little country store. We were having this discussion about our marriage, why he was refusing counseling or refusing to work to save it. This discussion was pretty intense but after we pulled into the store, the conversation stopped.

I was sitting in a Jeep truck and the window was open on my side. Suddenly out of the clear blue it felt like somebody grabbed a hold of my ear and pulled it all the way down to the seat. It hurt like hell. I mean I was like UHH! Whupped out! Jimmy looked at me and he goes, "What's wrong?" I said, "Something just pinched my ear and my head went down to the seat." I never knew a spirit could make you have a sensation like that.

Anyway, my ex asked me a question. I no longer remember what I answered but whatever it was, I said it in his grandfather's words.

136

Jimmy just knew it! And he goes, "Omigod, he used to always grab all us kids that way! We'd be going by him lickety-clippety, he'd grab our ears and he'd pull on 'em and we'd come to a dead halt. And it would hurt so bad."

All of a sudden it occurred to me I could say stop, so I said stop. Right away my head came back up and my ear did not hurt. Imagine. Jimmy asks me, "What does he have to say to me?" So I started telling him some things. Out of my mouth came the words, "This is like throwing pearls before swine." Apparently his grandfather was a doctor but he was also a strong Methodist and he used that expression all the time. Then this spirit that was talking through me made some comment about marriage but I couldn't quite get what it was he was saying. I felt like him pinch my ear again. I said no. And with that my hand went up from my lap.

My hand flew up and my wedding ring, which was on my hand, flew out the window. Now please, I'm in the passenger seat. I'm saying this ring went from my finger on my left hand up and out the right-hand window into the mud beside the truck. When that happened, Jimmy, my ex-husband went, "Ah, he's telling me I'm throwing the marriage down the drain into the mud." He went out and around and he found the ring in a mud puddle by the car. It wasn't hard to figure out where it was. But that ring literally went off my hand, across my body, out the open window and into the mud.

When I interviewed Jocelyn, she was just 19 but already she had had many psychic experiences. After a school friend of hers died, she asked for a sign of the girl's continuing presence. What she ultimately received was tiny but remarkable.

My sophomore year in high school there was a girl who died. Her name was Angie and she was like the most beautiful girl, you couldn't say a bad thing about her. She was just the nicest girl you'd ever met, completely like an angel—and her name was Angie.

She died on her way to work. She went around a corner, she was going too fast, she flipped her car upside down in the water and she drowned, she couldn't get out. My boyfriend at the time, he really loved her too. They used to ride the school bus together and she was one of his favorite people. When I had to call and tell him Angie had died, he was really upset.

About a month later, he called and bragged, "Me and my friends were going about a hundred down Clear Lake Road," which was the road where she had died. I was just so mad, I expressed this to him. How could he *do* this right after Angie had died that way? I would talk to her a lot saying, "Just take care of him, make sure that he's safe." It was around dusk, not quite dark, not quite light. My eyes were closed but this orange sensation, an orange light just glowed all the way around my room and I opened my eyes and it wasn't coming from anywhere. I felt that everything was gonna be okay, that she was going to take care of him.

Then time went on and he kept doing his stupid boy racing things. I would talk to her every night and say, "Angie, just make sure that he's safe—and if anything does happen, just be there with him so he's not alone." And then I felt silly. She was such a great person, such an angel. I felt like maybe I was just doing all this for me so I said, "Angie, why don't you give me something that I know only you would give me, something that I could actually hold." And the very next day in the car I'd completely forgot about what I'd asked her to do. And my mom picks up this penny—I wish I had brought it—and she says, "This is yours." And I said, "This isn't mine," and I didn't even look at it. I knew I didn't have any money in the car. She says, "Well, it's not mine. Did you look at it?" And I looked and it was a penny with an angel punched out in the middle. There was a hole in the penny. And I said, "This must be a customer's, mom. I've never seen it before." She says, "Well it's clearly not mine. I've never seen it either." And she insisted that it was mine.

Once I really looked at it, I started to laugh and said, "Well this must be from Angie." I usually wear it on my gold chain with an emerald cross my mom gave me. And everybody always says, "Where did you get that?" And I say, "An angel gave it to me."

Elizabeth is a highly intelligent woman who emigrated from Hungary to the United States with her husband in the early 1960s. When after many years her marriage ended and she had to decide on a new way of life, the spirit of her adoptive mother used forceful, though not violent, means to determine her choice of a new career.

For three years I kept thinking that I am an intellectual, right? I'm going to go to the university and pick up a degree. What am I going to do with that degree? I was 49 and there were already young

people with a couple of degrees working at McDonalds in management. So what am I going to do? A 49 year-old woman with an
accent. People don't consciously think that way. People are good and
people are kind—but it's built into the subconscious. Everyone
knows I'm a foreigner.

So I think my mama may have been steering me into hairdress-
ing. I had dreams, complicated dreams. In one of them she had an
awful wig with beautiful hair under it, but even the hair under it was
greasy and dirty and unkempt and I gave her a shower and then she
looked so much better.

Still I was studying reiki [*an Asian therapeutic practice*]. I had
completed first degree and I was getting ready to take second degree
initiation. Third degree is when you are able to teach others. Due to
the urgings of a strong-minded friend, I was going to get into reiki
mastership and I was going to be the big healer. [*Laughing sarcasti-
cally*] Anyway the time comes for the second degree initiation and I
go for my checkbook—it's $500. I go for the checkbook and I don't
have the money. I keep looking at the numbers and I can't find the
money. Two days after initiations were over, I found the money. I got
my bank statement and the money had been there all along. That day
I went down to the beauty school and signed up to become a
beautician.

Chris is a soft-voiced, confident woman who for many years
worked in management for the phone company. Soon after Chris's
mother died, she found a striking way to reach out to her family.

Mom was living with me then. When she passed away, it was 2
o'clock in the morning. I called my brothers and sisters to let them
know this had happened. My sister Laurie came over. After she'd
said her good-byes to mom in her bedroom, she walked into the living
room and picked up a picture. It was a picture we'd taken when my
mother, my sister and her family and I went to Disneyland. Laurie
was holding it and saying it was her favorite picture of the two of
them.

After a few hours we went up to my sister's home because the
kids were gonna be waking up. Stephanie, the granddaughter, woke
up and came downstairs. She didn't even look around. She just said,
"I had a dream about Grandma and going to Disneyland." We all sat
there kind of shocked because we knew what had happened about

the picture. We just kind of believe that it was my mother saying good-bye to her granddaughter in a very personal, unique way.

As I went through my notes about symbolic events, I noticed that almost all the reports I'd collected were from women. When men experience extraordinary coincidences or other hard-to-explain events, they seem reluctant to see symbolic meanings in them. Wayne told me of losing two symbolic objects while on an emotionally charged hiking trip. Only one of these events, he thought, might have been a healing gesture from the woman to whom he felt deeply tied for almost 30 years.

I'll start by saying I'm a skeptic. That's my natural bias though I probably have a different view of death than a lot of people. I worked as a surgical intensive care technician for about eight years and then I worked as an emergency department technician for another eight years, so I have plenty of experience around death. I view it more as a passage than a lot of people do, a passage rather than an ending. My skeptical side will say that's because I had to in order to keep dealing with it but I don't know that that's true.

Carol committed suicide after a long battle with illness. We had been partners for 13 years, then even after we started seeing other people, we'd still see each other two or three, four times a week. The life we had led together was so intense and we were so intertwined that I always felt the presence of her in my life.

After her death, I had to move into her house for a while to take care of her animals. Everything in there reminded me of her—of her presence, but also her absence. She'd wanted to be cremated. A couple of months ago I organized a trip to take her ashes up and spread them on a nice big granite slab in the mountains. Much of our sense of our shared spirituality came from the mountains, the high Sierras where we backpacked every year we were together, one summer as much as 64 days. That was where we focused our spirituality.

She loved to camp on these huge granite slabs in the Sierras. Sometimes in the glaciers they're smooth as glass. I found a place in a location that her mother and family could identify. A very close friend of Carol's and mine joined me and helped spread her ashes. I think I felt a sort of release at that time, not just with the spreading of the ashes but with the return to the Sierras. We always felt most at home there. So Carol was back home and I didn't have to tend to her. Two things of mine disappeared while I was on this trip.

The first was my balaclava, it's like a ski mask. In the Sierras, every morning you put your gear out in the sun on the granite so the frost will melt and the moisture will dry out in the sun. That was amongst them. I had my down coat, my down pants and my sleeping bag and my mattress, all these things out being dried on the granite. And I didn't leave camp. I sat in camp and cooked my only really hearty breakfast of the trip. When I got ready to go off on a day hike that afternoon, that balaclava was gone. Absolutely gone. And it would have stood out, dark blue on white granite. It hadn't blown into the lake, there hadn't been any wind. We didn't see anybody for six days, it was flat-out gone. If a deer had come by to eat it, my dog would've raised a fuss. Losing it wasn't life-threatening 'cause I had a down hood on my jacket. Still I searched absolutely everywhere for two days that we were there, in every crack and every piece of granite. My friend and I, we attributed it to "the granite ate it" or "the spirits ate it" or whatever. And it never reappeared, it's a total mystery.

I asked Wayne if he sensed any symbolic message in this disappearance. No, he told me, he didn't—even after I pointed out that his face mask might signify cutting himself off from the outside world. Carol's spirit, in taking it, might have been pressing him— as spirits often do—to open himself more to new experience, to get on with his life. "It wasn't like a memento or anything of that sort," he said, "but there was something else."

The last day of the trip, I smoked a little marijuana. The pipe and the backup pipe I had were Carol's, and they were in a little sheepskin coin purse that was Carol's. On the last night we were camped there, it was kind of cold and crisp so my friend and I, we built a fire. We sat around it, away from our tent, and smoked a little marijuana. We left some of our stuff around the fire: our cookset, so we could cook in the morning.

Well, it started hailing that night and hailed all night, until in some places there was a foot of hail on the ground. We had to pack up in the morning and get out. We looked and looked and cleaned up everything as we always do, very compulsively and meticulously. It's easy to do because you have only so many things, and they stand out like crazy in the woods. And after coming home, I could not find that coin purse with the pipes in it. And I racked my brain. Where could it be? And went through everything in my pack.

We finally decided that we left it by the campfire area. We picked up everything else around it, but because it was in a white sheepskin little purse and it was covered with hail, we had missed it. And I felt that there was kind of a connection with Carol. That this was something I needed to return to her. This was left in a meadow of hers, back out in the woods, and it freed me. It was sort of a freeing of having Carol still so much a part of my life. It got left in a good place that we'd been to many times, and it didn't have my name on it, thank goodness. *[Laughs]* So maybe somebody'll find it. Hopefully not. Maybe it'll wash out in the spring floods and never be found again. But, boy, it sure made a difference in my feeling. It had more of an impact than spreading her ashes. This was something, it felt like, I returned to her.

John, 65, is a retired journalist, photographer and teacher. Like Wayne he told me of a moving experience he hesitated to define as paranormal.

My grandfather was a preacher and I was sort of his namesake. He died when I was 15 or 16. About 20 years after he died, I was teaching photography in Los Angeles and I'd given this assignment to everybody. I said, "Go out and find a photographer you're interested in. Study their works and come back to talk to us about their things." So came the day for this and I'm sitting in this fairly small classroom and this one student has a portrait photographer she's interested in. And she passes the pictures around. . . . It's hard for me to talk about this. It's sort of an emotional thing.

The pictures come around and suddenly I'm looking at a picture of my grandfather. And I couldn't deal with it. I'm 35 or something like that—in this totally alien atmosphere. And suddenly I'm looking at an almost life-sized photograph of him. And I wasn't free enough to say, "My god, this is my grandfather." And he's looking right at me. I must have acted strange.

I didn't say to her, "I'd really like this photograph." I just couldn't deal with it, I just covered up. I still can't talk about it very easily but it shook me to my core. And afterwards I thought, was this maybe a way for my grandfather to reach me or something like that? Or, maybe it was the craziest coincidence in the world. But the fact was that it meant so much to me, I couldn't deal with it emotionally.

By contrast, women will often sense spirit communication coming to them via small, seemingly unremarkable events. One of my informants noted that on the June day when her father was buried, in front of his house, scraggly little rhododendron bushes which had never bloomed before showed a few blossoms for the first time. Her story recalled a comment made by Dr. Conant, the psychologist who interviewed recently widowed Massachusetts women in depth. One of them, she reported, "saw her husband's flowers blooming on special occasions as a sign from him."

A young interviewee of mine told me how, soon after her girlfriend was born, her girlfriend's mother, Char, was thinking about her own deceased father and thinking how much he would have enjoyed knowing his little granddaughter. All of a sudden, my interviewee said, "the blinds in the room started to go up and down, like someone was taking their finger and making them go up and down. And Char just knew that that was her dad waving." Other women reported having sensed loving messages in sunsets, rainbows and cloud formations. In the literature of the paranormal, rainbows are often mentioned as signs of contact with the dead.

In the next four accounts, the perceiver's sense of paranormal communication was heightened by a sequence of events. When I spoke to Melissa, she had had two intensely vivid dreams of her departed soulmate. Twenty years before, while she was in college, she had worked in a bar where Scott played in a band. Immediately after she had one of these dreams, she recalled a song connected with her lover that she hadn't thought of for a very long time.

> He had died of cancer and I went to visit him before he died. He couldn't speak because the cancer was in his throat but he wrote on pads and he told me in that dream that he was sorry that he couldn't have spoken to me with words but he had loved me very much. It was very comforting.
>
> That same day I woke up and I was feeling so wonderful that I'd had a communication with Scott and all of a sudden this song popped

into my head that he used to sing in the bar where we met. I hadn't thought of that song in like 15 years and I *knew* that he was sending me that song. The actual singing in my mind was not his voice but it was interesting because it's called "Dixie Chicken" and it goes, "You be my Dixie chicken, I'll be your Tennessee lamb and we will be together down in Dixieland." Which I took to mean that he was saying that when I die we'll be together. It was wonderful, really wonderful. I felt his presence very much that morning.

Sharon is a confident, multi-talented woman whose story of feeling her late husband's touch—and the major decision she made as a result—is reported in Chapter 7. For some years, she has been happily remarried. Her first husband, an officer in the Naval Reserves, died in a crash of a large navy plane where he was a flight attendant and loadmaster. Some months earlier, he made a point of purchasing life insurance. A string of unusual events relate to this policy.

For the year before he died, he had a premonition. First he thought he was gonna lose his dad. Then one day he came home and he says, "It's not dad, it's me." He went to the Christmas concert and they were singing the Hallelujah chorus from Handel's Messiah and all of a sudden something came over Ben and he went rushing out of the auditorium into the hallway. Fortunately his friend that he team taught with was near him. When he got home he was very shaken about it. He said, "I couldn't see. I was blind. I was banging into things and I was overwhelmed by this spiritual situation and I didn't know what to do." And Dave, his friend, came up to him and kind of embraced him and his sight came back. Whether he had a simple physical seizure, I don't know. He was checked out and nothing was wrong with him.

He insured himself with a pretty hefty insurance policy and when he left on the trip he said, "The policy's going to come due again in December. If I'm not back, if the flight is delayed in some way and I don't get back by the time it rolls over, I want you to renew it." I said, "Ben, that is really an expensive policy, I don't want to do that. We need the money for other things." He said, "Look, I haven't asked you very strongly to do many things in our marriage. I want this done." Okay.

So when he left, he left a letter tucked in our insurance folder. So that when I did open it, I would find it. So here's this big thing on a legal tablet, handwritten out, and it starts out, "I realize this is a really hard time for you, this is a crappy time for me to check out, but it was in order. I tried to take care of as many things as I could ahead of time." I went through all the stuff about what he wanted for the farm, for the children, how he hoped things would be handled financially. He knew he was going and he wrote this long missive to me.

Now the funny thing is, that letter disappears occasionally, then it pops up again. I keep thinking one of my kids is doing something because they know of the letter and I've shown it to the eldest. I went to get it to show to my son and it wasn't there. I asked my daughter about it and she says she doesn't have it. It's been twice that I've— it may just be my ditsy brain—that I've mislaid it somewhere. But I never had it out because I've very happily married and my first marriage is not something I deal with.

Allegra is an attractive lawyer in her thirties who works in an environmental field. The widow of a noted poet and herself gifted with a poet's eye, she mourned him for years. Then she developed a serious relationship with another man.

Since I got together with Liam, black sequins have been showing up. There's one, I can't remember where it was but it was in the bedroom. The second or the first one was right beside the bed. One was on the counter in the bathroom. One, I was making love with Liam and he found it on my chest, on my breastbone, right in the middle. We'd see each other on weekends. I thought they came with him, in some of his stuff, out of his bag, they were just falling. I asked Liam, I asked my brother. Nobody had any recognition of them and I didn't either. I don't know of any garments I've ever had with black sequins. Or purses or anything.

The first one I saw gave me a strong reaction, like presence. And black. Black is about death and transformation and introversion and isolation and something scary. [*Laughs*] And shiny sequins to me are like fish scales, they're tissue of a fish.

I'm a Pisces and my future husband is an avid fisherman. And fish is also Christ, and fish is feeding the multitudes. It's tremendously symbolic. And also the last sign of the zodiac, the turning of the cycle, the changing of the times. The millennium.

So sequins make me think fish scales, and black makes me think deep spiritual stuff that's like hazardous if not done correctly. We have so few rituals. It's dangerous in these times. But then a sequin is kind of a joyful thing too, it's celebration clothing. The first one I saw, it was like, "Whoa, where did this come from?" There was one after Liam was gone out of town and everything was lonely, still I woke up in the morning and it was between the bed and the door to my room, right in the middle of the walkway on the white carpet. Go figure. I'm clueless.

Allegra is a survivor of childhood sexual abuse. When I asked Allegra if she sensed any message in the sequins, this fact had some bearing on her answer.

I suspect that there is a spirit. When I think of it that way, I see kind of a catlike woman, very black, very sleek, very mobile, very bright, very purposeful, that is trying to talk to me about anger—because all my life I've suppressed anger completely so it's very dangerous for me. She's trying to get me past the rigidness that goes to paralysis/resentment kinds of things and into mobility—into using my anger for creative change.

Perri has had several loving, symbolic experiences with the spirit of her father. In life he was troubled, often angry and alcoholic. His daughter theorizes that, because he became a fighter pilot when he was just 19, he learned early to be macho but not to be gentle. Then, when Perri was 41, her father died suddenly of a massive heart attack. They never had a chance to say good-bye. About a month after he died, she sensed his presence under circumstances that had special significance for her.

I was meeting a friend in Philadelphia. I had a rental car and I was to meet her in a bus station downtown, then we'd take the bus together somewhere. Well, I ended up getting lost and the bus station's in a really scary neighborhood. I'm kind of a wimp and it was getting to be dark. Underground parking with no light, very scary. I had all these little encounters that made me fearful. So I finally got inside the terminal. I just wanted to sit down and relax a little bit and the only place there was a McDonalds. And I don't like McDonalds. I thought, how weird that's the only thing there.

My dad loved McDonalds. His dad had been a chemist who invented a preservative that keeps white bread. We used to have big fights over that when I was young. Anyhow, I went in there and I was just sitting there, exhausted. And then I have never had this happen before but it felt like his presence came to me. First it came like in a wind. I sort of thought what in the world is that? Then it felt like un-liquid rain. It felt like it was right above me and it just *poured* over me. And I just sobbed. And it was him, there was no mistaking. It was kind of funny, sitting there in McDonalds—but it was also very protective and loving.

Years later, she sensed contact with her father again under circumstances that recalled their shared delight in music.

I was the only one in the family that played the piano. My dad would come and sit in the living room. That was one of the few times he'd calm down and be so sweet and loving, when I played the piano. Sometimes he'd get teary eyed, he could be very sentimental.

After my mom passed on, he remarried. When he died, my stepmother lived in their house for a few years. After she moved out, my sister and I had to go over there to go through all my dad's papers and things. We'd work hours and hours and, of course, I had him on my mind. One night I came into the house to meet my sister but she wasn't there and it was dark and the lights wouldn't turn on for some reason and it was a little bit spooky for me. The next thing that happened is I heard music, music from a music box. At first I was overwhelmed. Then after I finally got the lights to turn on, I found it was a little piano music box that my dad had given me. That's what was playing. It was in a little pile of my old things I hadn't yet claimed. Seemed like it turned itself on.

I've thought about this over and over. I mean it could have been overwound, something could have bumped it. I guess it could be scientifically explained. But it falls so much in line with everything for me .... As if he was saying, "Here, don't forget to take this," or maybe just "I'm with you."

On another occasion, the sight of a wildly running horse conveyed to Perri what she believed was an important message from her father. In the next chapter we'll look at this and many other cases in which the actions of animals and birds have taken on important meanings for the people who saw them.

12

Animal Stories

LIKE MUSIC, horses were an interest that Perri shared with her father. "Horses and pianos," she told me, "were my healthiest connection to my dad." When she was trying to decide whether or not to buy a particular house, she sensed that her father was advising her.

I tend to be really tight fisted but I felt that it would be a smart move because I needed more space and I didn't want to take anything from my husband. I was thinking about using money that I had just inherited from my dad. I had to make the decision in one day because other people wanted the house. It was out in the country.

Okay, so I was walking through this house just thinking. I had dad on my mind a whole lot. I kept thinking, "Is this the right way to use this money?" and "What would dad think?" So then I went out on the balcony, and outside a neighbor's horse had gotten into the field of this house and it was running. It was a beautiful bay horse. The kind that my dad and I used to ride. A beautiful brown bay horse, just running wild. Head up, mane flying, tail up. And about a year before my dad died, I'd given him a sculpture of a horse that looked just like that in a running position.

So then I went back inside and I was still trying to figure things out. And then, like that rain I told you about earlier, something came pouring through me. This time it wasn't like from over me, it was in my body. It felt like a river of energy—and it was *music*. It was piano music and it probably lasted, oh, two or three minutes. But it was so powerful.

149

So that decided me. I bought the house and I have had no regrets. I just love it. It's my haven and my soul place.

Something similar happened when another woman I interviewed lost her husband, Mark, after a long battle with cancer. Right after he died, his sister-in-law who lived several hundred miles away, looked outside her window and saw a deer loping across her snow-covered lawn. She and her husband had lived there for 15 years. Never before had they seen a deer in their neighborhood, let alone crossing their property, so she thought that Mark might be sending them a message. She told his widow that maybe "he had sent the deer to let them know that he was free and happy."

Like deer, birds and butterflies are common symbols of freedom. Several people I interviewed had had after-death contacts that involved winged creatures. In Chapter 8, Connie described how, after the death of her daughter, a hummingbird perched on her hand and lingered there. Tim's parents lived over a thousand miles away. Soon after his father died during the night of a heart attack, Tim and his wife sensed a message in the actions of an unusual bird.

That morning we were sitting in the living room, just sitting there staring out, and a bird appeared on our porch that we'd never seen. It was yellow, a small yellow bird with a bit of black on it. And my wife and I just sat looking and looking. We both immediately thought the same thing, that my father loved to fly and if he was going to come say good-bye to me now, that would be what he'd do.

That bird stayed all morning. Whereas usually a bird'll come, flit around, eat something and be off, it was there till I left on a flight to go back home. Both my brothers were back there with my mom already. I felt like he'd come out to say good-bye to me.

My father was crazy about flying. His idea of a vacation was to get on a plane and get as many ups and downs as he could. If he flew from Chicago to California he'd have 30 stops along the way so he could go down, take off and land again. He flew whenever he could. I felt like finally he was getting to fly on his own. And I was talking to him, like he was actually there.

I flew home for about a week. About a week after that, I was sitting on the couch again, just kind of in a daze thinking about my dad, and the same type of bird was out in the tree again. Those are the only two times I've ever seen that specific bird.

When Alice spotted a kingfisher in an unlikely place, she sensed a greeting from a gracious lady.

A very special bird to me is the kingfisher. There's something about them I find very attractive. My dad's sister was like my Auntie Mame. Her name was Aunt Eve. One time when we celebrated my parents' fiftieth, she came out here to visit. We went to the High Desert Museum and Eve, who had a lot of money, led us all into the gift shop. They had all these little cloisonné birds and she asked all the women in our party to pick out a bird and she bought us each a bird. So I picked out a kingfisher and told her it was my favorite bird.

When she died, my dad and I went back to Ohio for her funeral. It was amazing because there was a whole aspect of her I didn't know. At her memorial service, there were hundreds of people from non-profit organizations. It turned out, she was a huge philanthropist.

So we were staying in this Marriott Inn on the Miami River which is a very Corps of Engineers, trashed river, all channelized and filthy. It's about the poorest excuse for a river I've ever seen still I went for my walk every morning along the bank of the river. And the first morning I went, a kingfisher emerged from the woods and flew along the river.

Now kingfishers don't hang around dirty water. You usually see them in the woods so it was pretty amazing to me. Maybe it didn't mean anything—but it felt like my Aunt Eve was showing up to me.

Soon after a death in the family, Grant and his wife sensed special meaning in the visit of an owl.

Last summer my wife's grandma passed away. She was 82 or so. The night before her funeral, I was outside in front of my house with Elaine's sister and her husband and an owl came down and swooped about two feet from me and went up into this tree right in our yard. It stayed there for three or four minutes. Elaine was in the house and Edith, who is Elaine's sister, went in and got her. The owl stayed in the tree until just after Elaine could go out and see and actually talk to it for a minute. Just kind of cooed, didn't ask it any questions, but I believe that it was Elaine's grandma.

Sure we have owls in the neighborhood but we rarely see 'em. It was pretty darn strange to have one that close and to have it stay even though people were moving around. We were just out there talking.... I thought it was Grandma Jean. Elaine had the same feeling. She had that feeling right away when she came out.

Eileen e-mailed me the following account. Soon after her husband's death, images of sea gulls—which had been dear to her husband—brought comfort to her and her family.

My first husband, Tom, and I were both very interested in the question of life after death and particularly the ability to communicate with the living, and we read a great deal on the subject. . . . Shortly before Tom's death from cancer, I asked him if he would try to stay around and give me support for a time. He said that he would if it was possible. When he lapsed into a coma, I was advised they could make him more comfortable with oxygen at the hospital. I went with him in the ambulance and my two daughters and son-in-law met me there. When the doctor said death would occur within the next two hours, we sent Ron, my son-in-law, home to bed as he had to be at work later that morning. After breathing ceased, we went to their house and Ron asked what time death had occurred.

Tom's favorite book of all time had been *Jonathan Livingston Seagull* and at a few minutes before 3:00 a.m. Ron heard the cry of a seagull climbing into the sky. We had never heard a gull cry at night before and he wondered if it was Tom's spirit ascending. As nearly as we could pinpoint it, the cry of the seagull rising into the sky must have happened very close to the time Tom's breathing ceased.

The following morning, my daughter was soaking in the bathtub and I called in to ask her if she had any stationery because I wanted to write a note to Tom's mother telling her about the seagull. Jan said the hair stood up on the back of her neck as she told me she had a pad of stationery in her purse—because she knew what I would find. The stationery had a field of blue across the top, with a white seagull in flight! I often feel this was a message of comfort and reassurance.

Joe reported an extraordinary death coincidence in which a butterfly landed on his hand.

I have a little sister who died of a brain tumor. I was sitting out in our yard reading, and I put the book down and I was watching this amazing sunset. I wasn't thinking about family, people that have died and aren't here any longer, but at the precise moment that my little sister died, I had a butterfly land on my hand.

It had a very calming effect on me but whether it was my dad or my little sister or my twin sister, whether it was related to any specific individual would be very difficult to pin down. I just interpreted it as an overall feeling of oneness—with reality, I guess you might call it. More of just a general "It's okay. These things happen."

Elisabeth Kübler-Ross has often written about butterflies as symbols of spirit survival. She tells us that, after World War II, she visited the Maidanek concentration camp and found, in the barracks where helpless prisoners spent their last nights before dying in the gas chamber, many drawings of butterflies on the walls. She speculates that the inmates who drew them must have been thinking that "soon they would leave their bodies the way a butterfly leaves its cocoon . . . that was the message they wanted to leave for future generations." It's easy to imagine, also, that some artists among them may have sensed their lost loved ones reaching out to them through the flutter of a butterfly—hovering close, perhaps even touching, despite the barbed wire that hemmed them in.

In Chapter 7, Joe told how at stressful times, he and his wife have often been comforted by smelling his late mother-in-law's favorite perfume filling the room around them. Joe was very fond of his wife's mother, Nancy, and has had many contact experiences with her, via differing routes. Here's how he described two vivid ADCs. The latter one involves a fox.

We were very close friends but it was at least half a year or longer after her death so she wasn't in my mind. I hadn't just been thinking about her or anything. It was Thanksgiving Day and we had had a typical Thanksgiving with family over and I had gotten tired so I excused myself from the crowd and went up to my bedroom to take a nap. While I was laying there, sort of in this presleep sort of state, I was suddenly startled awake by her standing at the foot of the bed. She looked to be at a much younger age and she was for all intents and purposes standing right there. It shocked me so much that I had trouble breathing. I mean it took my breath away. And she just said, "I'm perfectly fine and everything's okay," and then she just faded away.

It left me with a very secure, sort of warm and fuzzy feeling but I remember being absolutely shocked by the whole thing because I had not expected it at all. Since that time there have been numerous other incidents that have occurred around her.

One of Nancy's favorite things in the whole world—it was sort of her totem—was the fox. She collected little fox statues, things like that. Now, it was a particularly trying time when I was helping my wife sort through some of her mother's belongings. The family had waited almost a year to deal with her belongings so it was kind of a heavy thing for us. This happened on our back porch where we put dog food out for raccoons. There's three or four raccoons that we're feeding, that've become friendly. We had just gotten home after sorting through Nancy's things, and standing in the middle of our back deck and looking at our glass door and eating the dog food was a red fox—which is beyond comprehension. I mean, they are so secretive and nocturnal, they don't go anywhere during the day. And this one was standing square in the middle of our porch in the late afternoon and eating the dog food as if it had not a care in the world. And we figured that that was a very strong message that everything was being done the right way.

The death of Dorothy's beloved daughter, Amy, left an aching void in her life. At Amy's funeral, held in a church where she and her daughter had both spent countless fulfilling hours, the odd behavior of a little gray kitten took on special meaning for her.

My other daughter and I saw it at the same time and she said, "Look at the kitten, it's Amy." The kitten went around the end of the pew, rubbed against her dad's legs, and headed on back out through the congregation. And everybody who saw the kitten said, "Did you see the kitten? It was Amy." The church was packed. There were over 300 people there and it holds 250 at the most and they'd already thrown the kitten out twice, they carried it out. But the doors were open because of the hot day it was—so the kitten came in another door. The kitten knew all the doors as if it was Amy. We all thought of Amy.

I've always thought of myself as a cat person. I grew up with cats and in the course of my adult life, I have been owned by three. I've always enjoyed other people's dogs but I never thought of living with one myself—until I started interviewing people about their ADCs. Dorothy's story of the kitten at her daughter's funeral is the most intense I collected about cats. But several of my 78 interviewees reported deeply emotional contact experiences with precious, departed dogs. Jocelyn sensed the presence of two different dogs she lived with at different times during her childhood.

When I was five, my mom and dad bought me this dog, Ginger, for my birthday. And I loved this dog. She was always close with my brother and I. She had this favorite blanket that she would hide underneath 'cause it was an afghan with holes and she could see 'cause she was a dachshund. She'd look at you, it was really kind of funny, and she'd play these games. One summer day, Ginger fell asleep in the car and died. I was eight at the time. Afterwards I quit eating, I quit talking. I would think about her and cry about her.

For about a year after she died, we never used the blanket 'cause it reminded us too much of her. Then one time my mom said, "Go, get it," and when I was walking up to it I saw these eyes in it. I saw Ginger's eyes and I got really scared and started to cry. My mom thought maybe I was imagining it. Then every year at Christmastime I always arranged the presents very neatly under the tree. One time, I had my back to the living room and no one else was around and I felt this poke like someone had taken their finger and poked me in the back. I turned around and looked and it was Ginger. I saw her just as plain as day and she was wagging her tail. I think she was trying to tell me that she was okay. She just wanted to say hi.

Then there was my dog Bud which I got probably when I was about ten. He was always very connected to us. I always felt like him and I knew each other from somewhere else. Then when he was seven or eight, he got sick with his kidneys and he was just gradually dying and wouldn't eat anymore so I knew we had to take him to be put to sleep. So I told Bud I just needed to know that this was the right thing to do. I wanted him to come back and tell me some way and show me that he was okay.

After he was gone, I would come home from school and I would just feel empty, coming home to a completely empty house. Maybe a week or two had passed and I was sitting, not really even thinking about Bud, just thinking how silent it was, and I heard him walk into the bathroom. Cause we had linoleum and I could always hear his paws when he'd walk into the bathroom and he'd always jump up on the toilet and drink out of it, and it's like such a distinct noise. I'm just sitting there and I hear him walk in the bathroom and I'm smiling and then I hear him drinking out of the toilet. And I just start to laugh and I start to cry. And I called my friend's mom and said, "I think Bud just visited me and he's happy, he's okay now."

Yona is an administrator with a child care program and teaches at a Jewish religious school. The day a dog of hers died, she sensed two remarkable death coincidences.

He looked like a police dog. He was a mixed Lab, black with those little tan markings over the eyes. I always thought that I was really good with dogs and I had just trained him but, no, it was really him, you know. He was just amazing. We would take him to the vet sometimes because he would have worms. In those days, that's what you did. My husband and I would be sitting there, just reading, and all of a sudden we'd look at each other because we could just feel the dog concentrating on us, like "Get me out of here!" I mean, we could both feel it at the same time. That's what he was like. He was the closest, most wonderful dog for communication in every way.

Well, I was going to community college then—twice a week and it was a long day. I'm out there, just studying and I'm sitting during the breaks. This was just about the time when my dog was being shot. He'd apparently got into some chickens and our neighbor had shot him with my friend there to see it—but I hadn't heard a word about that yet. I'm reading history about the Native Americans, what happened to them. And I started crying. I thought, "This is really crazy." I'm an emotional person but this is really crazy.

Then later on, like four or five hours later, it was getting to be almost sunset. I went up onto the hill to go to my class and all of a sudden I got this incredible feeling of release and liberation and joy. I just had to run. It felt so good. And then when I got home that night and found out what had happened, it was all really clear to me. I did not grieve as much as I would have if I hadn't already had both of those experiences.

It was such a traumatic thing, my dog being shot. I mean, my dog was there when my son was born. It was really a big deal. But it was like I was being carried by a wave, the emotions that went through me! It was like, "Wow, where did this come from?" I'm just sitting there quietly, just studying and feeling pretty good, and these things just came over me. So when I found what had happened, I was really okay. I felt like I'd been given a gift by my dog. I mean, there's nothing I could do. And he'd been released. I had never thought of a dog being released. It wouldn't have been in my belief system to have said anything like that about a dog. It was just that I experienced it before I knew. This dog was a phenomenal dog.

Charlie P. is an artist in his thirties who works in a glass foundry. When a favorite dog of his died almost 3,000 miles away, he sensed its passing.

The dog's name was Happy, Happy Dog. Half whippet, half beagle, really fast, a beautiful dog. It still lived in New York with my mom and I was living here in Oregon and one night I had a dream with Happy Dog in it. Never before had a dream with Happy Dog in it. And she turns and she has a skeleton face. That's all I remember from that dream. And when I wake up I put two and two together real quick: Happy Dog just died. And she did. I got it in a letter shortly afterwards that week.

Summer, the dance teacher quoted at length in Chapter 2, told me this extraordinary story about two heroes: a soldier in Vietnam and his beloved dog. A friends of hers in San Antonio, Texas—a golf pro—shared this experience with her.

Bob said, I was in Vietnam and I was in the thick of a firefight in the jungle and I was with like a dozen guys and they were in the jungle and all of a sudden they received a direct hit. Several of his friends were killed outright. He was badly wounded, a head wound. Blood started flowing down into his eyes and he got lost. He was calling out to his friends but he couldn't find anyone. All of a sudden his dog, Rusty, was right in front of him, a little cocker spaniel, and Rusty was jumping up and down and barking.

This was his dog from home, an old dog. Bob's childhood dog—he was raised with this dog all through middle school and teen age. And Bob said, "It was just real clear to me. He was barking and when I went to pet him, he ran off down the trail right ahead of me and kept barking and was leading me down the trail." He couldn't see because of the blood in his eyes but that dog stayed right in front of him, barking. He led him right down the trail and Bob staggered back to a headquarters.

As soon as he came into the clearing, they rushed up and put him on a stretcher and took him to the hospital. He was in the hospital two weeks and then—what was it Vietnam guys call it?—that was his "ticket home." He had a bad enough wound to go home but he's not disabled or anything.

So he came home, got off the plane at San Antonio, hugged his mom and relatives, and as soon as they had their first round of hugs, he said, "How's Rusty?" And his mom said, "Well son, I didn't want to tell you but he died of a heart attack, he didn't suffer or anything, he died suddenly." So Bob said, "When?" And it was the *date* and *time*. And Bob always will believe that his dog died of a heart attack when he was wounded.... *[For a moment stops talking, in tears.]* Died of a heart attack when he was wounded and then went to save him.

"That's real love," I said. And Summer responded, "Real love. They could teach us a few."

Often visits from the spirit world are helpful gifts. In the next chapter we look at more of them.

13

More Help and Guidance from Loving Spirits

CINDY TOLD US ABOUT TWO INCIDENTS where spirit guidance may well have saved lives. The first one happened to her sister-in-law.

> She was driving with my two nieces and nephew in the car. They live up in the interior of British Columbia and it gets very icy up there. Well, the tires caught the ice and they went over a cliff about two stories high. My little niece was probably around five then. It started with her saying this, but afterward all three of the kids agreed that their grandmother, who had passed away, said, "Get your head down, get your head down. Relax, get your head down." The whole time they were going over the cliff. And they all walked away without a bruise.

The second incident involved Cindy herself on the day when a disturbed teenager shot up the Springfield, Oregon school her son attended, killing 2 and injuring another 22.

> My kids, both of them went to Thurston High School and my husband said they totally were protected by a guardian angel. Cause that day we were one minute late, literally. My son is usually in the hallway with Ryan Atteberry [*who was shot in the face*]. Him and Ryan are really good friends. They always meet in the band room. My son had his trumpet in hand and the school door was open and the police officer that was in front of us ran over and said, "Back in the

159

car! Take your kids, go!" You know, we were the first in behind him, behind the police officer.

It's weird why we were late. I knew my dad was going up to Portland. I had asked him if he needed eggs—cause I keep chickens—and he goes, "Well, I don't really need them until I come back." But the day of the shooting, about two days early, I decided I'm gonna take them in to work and put them in my fridge there. It's like I stopped the car in the driveway, got out, went in the house, got the eggs out of my kitchen fridge, came back out to the car—and that's exactly how late we were. Otherwise my son would've been with Ryan in the hallway. So in my husband's philosophy, somebody was watching out for him.

Cindy, the daughter of a psychic mother, was one of my most interesting informants, a very sensitive woman who has had many paranormal experiences. The first year after her mother died, Cindy dreamt of her almost every night. Often in those dreams, her mother gave her advice.

My daughter was six when my mom passed away. And they had a real bond, just an incredible bond. When Heather was having so much trouble handling the fact that her grandma had died, mom would come to me in dreams and say, "Just be patient. This is what she's going through right now." She'd come to me and say, "She doesn't want to tell you all that she's feeling, because she doesn't want to make you cry." You know, she was almost like a counselor. I wouldn't have a clue but she'd say things. The next day I would get up and it was like, "Okay, I'm going to look at it more from this perspective." And that really helped.

You kind of wonder. How would I know something in a dream if obviously during the day I didn't know that? People say it's your subconscious, that your thoughts relax or whatever when you sleep and you see things you're too stressed out to see during the day. But it never felt that way to me.

Do visitors from the other side truly give advice? Tom is one of the many informants who told me yes, they do. After his wife died in an accident, her spirit seems to have taken a helpful interest not only in Tom's welfare but in that of her best girlfriend.

Norma's girlfriend recently had a separation from her live-in boyfriend of eight years and then to lose her best friend right afterwards, that was pretty rough on her. But she said that one night, she woke up in the middle of the night. There was a river in her dream and Norma was standing on the other side, and she said Everything will be okay. Forget about this guy. Don't be in a big hurry to find someone else but things will be all right. "I wanted to talk to her," [Norma's girlfriend] said, "but she just talked to me and said that."

Then when I was looking for my wife's insurance papers, I *could* not find her birth certificate. I knew that she had a birth certificate in this little box. And I went through that box twenty times and I was really getting stressed. It's like you're on a roller coaster and you want somebody to just press the stop button but you can't. I was really getting frantic and I said, "Norma, where did you put that birth certificate?" She said, "It's in that box, just keep looking for it." And I swear, the next time there it was, right where she said. So I said, "Thank you." And she said, "I told you so."

Charlie's mother made her transition a few years ago. For a while after her death, when he couldn't find something, he would ask her help.

For example, I was going to get out the birthday candles. I was going to put some birthday candles on a cake and we had no clue where the candles were. So I went out in the kitchen and I said, "Mom, help me find the candles." And she says, "It's over on this side of the kitchen." And I was looking up and she says, "No, it's not up above, it's down below." And then she says, "It's in the drawer. Not that drawer, the next one." And I went right to it and opened it and there they were. That happened many times.

Now I will say that a couple times it didn't work. But it did work a lot of the time. So it was way beyond chance.

Sometimes help from the spirit world can just take the form of a reassuring, seemingly physical gesture. In the following two cases, the touch of a loved one's hand helped the perceiver at a crucial time. When Christina was in her early twenties, her life was at a turning point.

I was really upset. It had to do with the breakup of a relationship I'd had for probably four years. And I felt that I was really stuck in my job in Portland. This was in the sixties and, you know, there was the revolution that was going on.

I woke up because I could feel somebody holding my hand. My old auntie who had lived with us. She said that everything was going to be okay. I didn't exactly hear this but I sensed it in my head.

So I went to work—I used to walk to work. It was a spring morning and a really nice day. And my gosh if it wasn't that same day I was taking the escalator down to the cafeteria in the new Georgia Pacific Building and I saw my cousin, Lars, and his friend, Jerry. And I said, "What're you doing here?" And they said they were planning to go over to the far side of the Cascades, to help build this cabin for Lars's dad. So they said, "Why don't you go with us?" And I thought, I have nothing to lose, everything to gain.

So I went in and gave notice. I didn't have any money to speak of and I was living with three other girls. You always had to share a room with somebody. So, yeah, I just said I was going. I told everyone I was going to live in a commune outside. And they said, "What are you going to do about money?" And I said, "Well, I won't have any money to worry about."

So I spent the summer with Lars and Jerry and this old man who was actually the contractor. And my girl cousin and her husband and their little boy. And it was wonderful, always. We just had such a great time. It was just because my old auntie had reassured me, I wasn't afraid to take the risk.

When Barbara was 31, she had major surgery and very nearly died. She credits her survival largely to the intervention of her grandfather's spirit.

The surgery was in the morning and that night when I came to, I remember rolling over. You know how you're in a hospital bed and there are those bars, metal things. I was on my right side and there was an IV in my right arm. And my arm was kind of through the bars. And what made me open my eyes was, somebody took my hand and it was my grandpa. And he'd died nineteen years before but we'd been very close.

Of course I was in a drugged state. Let's face it, I'd had general anesthesia that morning. But I knew who it was because he wore the same kind of pin-striped suit. And it smelled like my grandpa—and I hadn't smelled anything like that for years! I looked up and he was smiling down. Then when our eyes connected, he put his other hand around my hand. He had a hand on top and a hand underneath my right hand and he gave it a very gentle squeeze. And he said, "It's going to be okay. Don't worry."

Two days later, they were giving me a bath. My GP just happened to be going by the door and he heard me say, "I'm starting to feel real funny." Dr. Schwartz whipped in. He took one look at me and I heard him hit the emergency button. He yelled at this poor little nurse assistant who was giving me a bath and said, "Go to the nurses' station and get me some ice cream ASAP!" He really yelled it. I jumped when he said it. Then he stood back and looked at me. He said, "You're going to have a test tomorrow. I think we've got stress diabetes."

Now six months earlier I'd been diagnosed with hypoglycemia so I thought he was out of his mind. But he was a wonderful doctor. That man could just *look* at somebody. . . . My glucose tolerance test came back and I tested out as a diabetic and he was sure it was stress diabetes. But what got me through it was Grandpa. He said it was going to be okay."

Barbara comes from a privileged and very distinguished background—but one where drinking problems have abounded. Parallel contact experiences saved both Barbara and her mother from bondage to the bottle.

My mother's father's family is in the *Almanach de Gotha*. I remember hearing someone in the family said, "We don't have alcoholics in *our* family." The problem is, while Mother and I are cousins of Prince Philip, her *mother's* people were descended from Samuel Adams, the patriot, and he was an alcoholic. What sobered Mother up was one time when she was praying and looking at a knotty pine ceiling, she saw her mother's face. And her mother was crying. She never took another drink.

The one time she materialized for me was not long after she died. I was praying for guidance, trying to figure out what to do with her things, with her estate. I was actually on my knees praying and she materialized on the other side of the room. And she said, "Barb, you've got to stop drinking." And I haven't had a drink since.

After Beverly lost her husband, she grieved for him painfully for years. On several occasions, he contacted her through dreams. The night before she received disturbing news, a dream visit from him reassured her.

On the anniversary of his death, I had a dream where I was waiting in front of a train, waiting for him to get off, and he didn't get off and he didn't get off. So I went into this boxcar and there was a man with a sheet over him and I started calling his name and then something clicked. I must've consciously remembered that he died, right there in my dream. I started to panic, I started yelling—and he suddenly sprang up and said, "I'm fine. You have to go back now and I have to stay here." And I got off the train.

It was a real brief dream. I woke up and I knew that he wasn't gonna come back anymore. That that was it. But I felt good, you know. When I woke up in the morning, I felt no sadness, I felt really good. Later on that day I found out that Mary, who'd been like a second mother to me since I was two, had passed away. And for some reason, it didn't destroy me. It was like he gave me back the final piece of my heart.

Anna received help from the spirit of another beloved woman named Mary after this woman died under particularly grisly circumstances. Mary was an elderly physician who ran a halfway house for recovering addicts; she and her husband Gabe lived on the premises. Anna was employed there as a social worker.

My mother is still alive but Mary gave me mothering so she was more than my boss, she was a mentor and a mother figure. There was a man that she'd asked to leave the house because he'd had sex with a woman there. This was a man who'd been in jail before and he was being treated for addiction. He called up and he threatened Mary and everybody at the house. I wanted to call the parole officer but she said, "No, this is a house of love. We won't call the police." And I felt not good about this all day long.

The next evening we had another threat. And as I sat with Mary I did something that I'd never done before which was lay my head in her lap and she stroked my head. I told her how much it touched my heart and how much mothering I received just from this experience. Sometime during the night this guy came in and he shot Mary and Gabe at point blank range. Then he took off in her car.

So the next morning as I was driving to work, I head the news. By the time I got there, the bodies of Mary and her husband were being hauled away. Doors and everything were broken in. The police had everybody outside. The people who'd been staying in the house were hysterical. Everybody was a wreck because these were fragile people already.

The police let me in. I walked into Mary's room and I saw the bloody sheets. When I saw them, I almost threw up. But there was a window behind me and at that instant, this ray of golden light came over my right shoulder into the room and down towards the sheets. And this peace came in. And I heard, "Don't make a scene. Just do what's meant to be done. Put 'em in the new washer." *[Laughs]* That was the first thing I heard. I heard it in my head but I heard it very clearly and there was definitely this golden light.

Once she had my attention, she made a *joke*. She says, "I guess from now on they'll call me Bloody Mary." Now her name was Mary but Bloody Mary's an alcoholic drink and she'd been in AA for forty years and working with alcoholics. So then I said in my mind, like "Where are you?" or "What happened?" or "What was it like?" It's like asking all these questions at once cause it was such a shock. And her answer to me. . . . *[chuckling]* She says, "You know, it was just like 'Beam me up, Scotty.' One minute I was asleep and the next minute I was with all my old friends."

I've never forgotten that image of it being like Beam me up, Scotty. It reframed my whole concept of dying. That was one thing. The second thing was that it gave me the strength for the next three days to do a whole lot of stuff. Everybody else was in drama and trauma and making big deals and fear and anger and everything else. I had to find places for people; I had to find places for the food. And I had to give away everything in the place to homeless shelters or whatever.

Then Mary's children came in from out of town. The killer had been apprehended but I had to help them, get them to the police and get them Mary's car. Tell them what had happened and get them the files. So I had a huge amount to do and that experience with Mary gave me the strength and the wisdom and the hope to go through the whole thing.

After Lisa found an odd old brooch in her home under mysterious circumstances, her housemate suggested that she see a psychic. Soon she received valuable advice through an unexpected route.

The psychic took the brooch, looked at me and she goes, "You're psychic. You take this home and you do automatic writing to find out about it. Someone's trying to tell you something."

So I went home and I sat there. I had never done automatic writing before. I said a little prayer. I called in my Higher Power, I called in Jesus. I called in angels, like "Protect me. If this is somebody dark, I don't want anything." So then I started to write. It was easy, it flowed....

One of the women that was talking gave me her name, it was Cara. Basically, she told me, "We're here for you." My whole life I always prayed for like world peace and stuff. I never prayed for material help. I was always on my own. She said, "But we wanted you to know that you can pray for physical things. You shouldn't be afraid of this." She was talking about, like the spirit realm that I was always resisting, all the things that I was always an open-minded cynic about. She was saying, "This is a world you should be comfortable in, not afraid of." So then I asked, "Is there anything else that you want to tell me?" And at that time, I was looking for a car because the car I had was practically dead. I had just looked at a car that day. And she said, "Don't buy any car right now. When the need arises, one will be provided."

So I was like, "What does that mean?" I had no history of anybody providing a car for me. But then a week or two later, I came home one day and my roommate said, "Your father called. He wants you to call him back. Something about a car. He said make sure you don't buy a car." And I was like, Oh my God. We weren't from the kind of family where ... we weren't ever given cars or much of anything else.

But anyway I called him back and his brother had called him and told him his friend was selling his station wagon. And then my father called me to see if I wanted *his* car. Which is really weird because that's what the automatic writing had said would happen. And I had no experience in my whole life that that would ever happen.

Roni is a vivid, multi-talented woman who has had two separate, very different careers—first as a nurse, then as a designer of spectacular costumes crafted of velvets and silks, some hand-painted or trimmed with beads. When she was a young nurse she formed a close friendship with an intern. After his premature death, she often sensed his help and advice.

One of my very best friends had a heart attack. He was an intern and I took care of him. The night before he died he was real stable. I was working 11:00 to 7:00 with him. Somehow we both knew this was good-bye night. We sat there and talked and talked. It was like beyond bonding, like a recognition and understanding of your life. A thing about it's okay to die, but nothing was ever spoken directly.

I could tell from the way the whole night went. It was quiet and peaceful. We'd talk about other things. I'd sleep, he'd touch me and I'd wake, then we'd talk again. When I left him in the morning, I had such a feeling of fulfillment. About 10 o'clock they called me to tell me he'd had a cardiac arrest and died and I went completely hysterical because he was the first person I can ever remember that just knocked me off my pins.

Dan was such a fabulous doctor and after he was dead, I'd be doing something and I'd be really scared—and I would just talk to him. I'd take a deep breath and I'd say, "Dan, am I doing this right?" It was like I could hear him in my head talking to me, helping me out, talking me through it. But at the time I didn't realize that's what was happening. I was just too young and too involved in other things. Still I knew that I had like this extra sense.

Roni continued to work as a nurse through her loving marriage to Kenny. She harbored a longing to switch professions, to work at some more artistic endeavor, but financial pressures prevented her from taking the risk. Then in 1988, her husband died in an accident.

I remember him saying to me one night in a dream, "I died so you could do whatever you want." I didn't realize what that meant for six months. Then in six months, my life was so drastically changed that then I understood the dreams.

Kenny was a teacher so I got his retirement. Because it was a car accident, it was double indemnity. So it was over $100,000, all at one time, and it made a big difference. I was able to take a whole year off of work. I went to the university for six months and got a little education in fiber and then decided that I'd start my own business. I can't believe I did that—but now my business is thriving.

Kenny still comes to me in dreams. I think he's visiting or he wants to make me aware of something. Usually it's about money. What happens is I'll be worried, worried, worried about money. I'll get frazzled about it and then that night I'll have a dream and it'll be Kenny and he's say, "Don't frazzle about it. Everything's gonna work out fine, the check is coming today." Or "You're gonna get money." And sure enough, it always happens.

Alan is an Englishman whom I interviewed via e-mail. A widower, he has sensed helpful messages from his late wife.

My wife died five years ago after a marriage of nearly 40 years. I have had vivid dreams in which she gave me advice, the value of which only became apparent some time afterwards. . . . Some time after she died, I had a vivid dream in which she suggested that I get to know a female friend of hers, a lecturer at the university where my wife taught. At the time I had only met this woman once. I took no notice for a long time, but I am now developing a serious relationship with her.

I find it impossible, whatever the psychiatrists say, to accept that my wife is "gone" and no longer exists in some form. It does not "feel" as if this has happened and I have heard this said by other people in a similar situation.

My brother-in-law's mother died at about the same time. Soon afterwards he had a premonition that prevented him from going to a place where a terrorist bomb exploded in a city centre. He thought it was a warning from his mother, but this was so far outside his usual experience that it frightened him.

I am agnostic at the moment over the meaning of such events. I do not share the psychiatric view that it all must be hallucinatory, but nor do I share the view of "believing" spiritualists, who seem to see "spirits" everywhere. Other explanations are possible. The idea of multiple universes is current in quantum physics, so that one could be picking up emanations from other universes in which the dead person is still alive.

When I first heard the following story, it brought me up short. I too can be skeptical about things paranormal. Nonetheless, the man who told me this holds a responsible job and was recommended to me by a wise and reliable woman.

When this happened, I was about 19 and into weight training. And I neither drank nor did drugs—to this day, the same thing. My brother and I were renting a house, my bedroom was in the front porch which was enclosed. We had just been to the gym, it was the middle of the day. We put our gym gear away and I laid down on the bed. It was one of those old style beds where they had kind of a wire mesh nailed to two-by-fours and they dropped the mattress on top of it. Maybe you'd call it a cot. Anyway, I laid down on the bed at about two in the afternoon. I laid down and I rose out of the bed. About two feet out of the bed. Levitated.

Well, the first thing I said, "I don't believe this." Kind of derisively. I heard a voice—I don't know the source of this voice or what was going on. I heard a voice that said, "You don't believe this?" And I said, "No." And they said, "Okay." At that point I fell onto the bed but I fell vertically *[in line with the mattress, in the normal position.]* I got a sarcastic, "You don't believe this?" and I said "No." And I rose up again but this time when I was levitated, I was turned diagonally. So I would be at an angle to the bed. Raised two or three feet. So when I fell I hit the wooden bars. It hurt but it didn't do any damage. This time pain showed me that it happened. I was not about to have that same experience again so I said, "I believe it."

And at the same time, someone is coming through the front porch windows, a total stranger, and I said, "What the heck are you doing here?" And he said, "I'm lost." Now there's no way he could be lost cause this is the front of the house, we're not on the road. And then he said, "Sorry," and got back down out of the windows and left. Within two seconds of me falling back on the bed and regrouping, this gentleman comes through the window. *[Laughs]* With some lame reason why he's climbing through my window. And I would've been asleep if this hadn't all happened.

Here's another story about apparent help from an unidentified source. While Elizabeth was trapped in a difficult marriage, with two small children, she sensed that she was receiving help from a friendly spirit in her rented house.

I was sewing everything my girls and I wore back then. And I was forever paranoid about leaving the scissors on the coffee table where the girls could find it and hurt themselves. One time I knew for sure I left the scissors on the coffee table and the girls were in the living room and I rushed out there and there were no scissors on the coffee table. I looked for those scissors for days and days. I asked the girls about it. "No, mommy," they said. There was a built-in bookcase in the living room wall and one day I went to take a book out from the very top shelf. I got a stepstool and reached all the way up. As I pulled out the book, the scissors fell down. I never put those scissors way up there.

It couldn't have been my husband either, he wasn't home at that time. There were the girls and I. I left the scissors on the coffee table and somebody, some *being* put them up on the highest shelf.

Another time I had an experience with a broom when I was sweeping the kitchen. It was around 11:30 at night and my husband was out with friends seeing a film. The babies were asleep, and I was exhausted. I'd been cleaning house and ironing and sewing. That was the last stroke, to clean the kitchen floor.

I swept up whatever there was to sweep up and I set the broom against the wall about three steps away from me, and I bent down to collect the paper and whatever with my hand. As I was looking up, I saw the broom standing up from the wall, *freestanding* within my reach. At the time the thought that someone is helping me ran through my mind. Let's do it together. I don't have to do the three steps over there to bring it back here. And there were times where I saw out of the corner of my eye that there were some coat hangers swinging on a doorknob and when I looked right at them, *just then* the coat hangers stopped swinging.

This last detail—about the seemingly instant response of a physical object to the perceiver's attention—sounded especially familiar to me. I myself have had experiences like that, and others have reported similar events. They tell you that an unseen presence is near, that it's aware of you and wants you to know this.

In time Elizabeth came to suspect that her ghostly companion was the dead son of her landlady, a young pilot who had committed suicide over his failed marriage to a Frenchwoman. In the next chapter we'll look at stories of other ghost presences—most of them not so agreeable.

14

Ghosts, Possession, and Things That Go Bump in the Night

NO ONE I'VE INTERVIEWED has ever been physically injured by a ghostly presence. Still a quarter of them have reported contacts with non-earthly beings to whom they felt no personal connection. A number have lived in haunted houses. In keeping with folklore, those houses often have a gory past.

Barbara and her husband bought a beautiful home in Southern California. It was a designer's dream, built in a square with a tree in the middle. "I was never afraid," she told me.

> But it scared the bejesus out of people because they would hear these noises, and doors would open and close, and they'd see faces. And they'd hear running up and down the halls. We found out later that the first owner was an artist who had had it built. And he had been having an affair with his model. And the wife shot the model, shot the husband, and then killed herself in that room. And I kept seeing this face in this hallway on the other side of the house from where the shooting was.

Jocelyn told me about a house where her parents and older siblings used to live.

When they were living in Massachusetts, they lived where a man had killed himself. My mom would lay in bed at night and hear him up in the attic walking, or hear his rocking chair. There wasn't any rocking chair up there still she'd hear him rocking or walking back and forth. He was really restless, he'd open and close the door a lot. And he'd close my brother and sister up there. A lot of times he would close the door behind them.

My dad never believed and one night my mom left him alone in the house with the two kids and he saw a man in the hallway. He was holding a lantern and he just looked at my dad like, What're *you* doing here? My mom says dad just bolted out of the house, took both the kids, came and got her and they did not go back to the house that night because he just could not deal with it.

While Jerry was working as a correspondent for *Life* magazine, he lived for a time in Madrid with his wife Jenny and their combined family of four children—her two daughters and his two sons from previous marriages. He went down to Ibiza in the Balearic Islands to open a house they'd rented for the summer.

I'd never been in it before. I lay down on the couch by the fireplace and I was awakened by a ghost. The first ghost I'd ever seen in my life. It was a Walt Disney type of ghost, you know. Right in front of the fireplace fluttering white. Well Jenny was a tremendously spiritual person, and not in the conventional sense. Spirits gathered around her. So when she came down with the kids the next day, I told her and she said, "Oh dear. We're going to drive the poor thing outside."

The next day after Jenny comes, we're all in the kitchen getting supper ready and suddenly there's a knock on the door. She said, "Will you answer that, sweetie?" and I said sure. No one there, you know. She said, "That's probably our friend, the ghost you saw last night. He'll probably go around, whoever he is, knocking on our windows." And sure enough he started off, right around the house— rap rap rap . . . rap rap rap—right around the house. It was incredible. She had an incredible spiritual quality about her. [*After Jenny's premature death, as reported in Chapter 3, Jerry had nightly visits from her for four or five years in which she advised him about raising their children.*]

Incidentally, in those days all the natives lived on one end of the island. All the Easterneros, all the foreigners, lived on the other end. The natives would come by to go to the grocery store and they'd always stare at our place. So one day I asked one of them, "Why are you staring?" And she says, "Well, your house is haunted." And I said, "What do you mean by that?" So she told us of a French painter, very well known, who was having a one man show in Paris. He left his wife in the house and she was a little off. There was a balcony on the roof. She'd get up there and she'd holler—cause it was an old Phoenician colony—"The Phoenicians are coming! The Phoenicians are coming!" And the natives got very scared so they called the cops. And the cops took her off to Barcelona and put her in an institution.

Well, the painter came home and found out where she was and went and got her. He brought her home and shot her and himself. Committed suicide. And they said the house has been haunted ever since.

From other stories Jerry told me about Jenny, she seems indeed to have had a natural intimacy with the paranormal. She could, for instance, as something of a parlor trick, entertain her children by making water glasses move across the dining table without touching them. Psychokinetic stunts like these were studied intensively by scientists in the old Soviet Union and more than once have been recorded on film.

When Jenny, Jerry and their family left Spain for California, they moved to a little house in Topanga in the Santa Monica Mountains. Jenny started working toward a doctorate in archeology at UCLA and, a few months later, gave birth to Amanda. When Amanda was about a month old, they noticed that the nightlight next to her crib seemed to have burned out. When they checked, they discovered that the light itself had disappeared. Six weeks later they found it stuffed under Amanda's mattress in her crib.

The same evening that the nightlight disappeared, something even weirder happened. Extending back from the headboard of their bed was a flat counter about 18 inches deep. There Jenny had piled a batch of her books and papers for school. Just as she went to turn off a lamp and come to bed, papers flew up from the pile on the headboard.

The whole room was just full of flying papers sailing around. I mean, it was so startling, it was incredible. Of course, nothing to her at all. She had some intuitive thing, I don't know what it was. But *me,* my God, all these things start flying around and you think, What's going on? All the windows were closed. The papers flew around for probably a minute and a half, two minutes. Books even came off the top. They didn't fly but they banged on the floor. I don't know what they were trying to tell us. Whether she shouldn't be going to school or what. But anyway. Things stopped flying around after a while so we finally got a chance to pick them up.

Then one night I woke up and there was a ghost at the foot of the bed. Jenny was sleeping beside me in the bed but she never woke up. The first time the ghost appeared, it was just exactly like the ghost in Ibiza—only much bigger. I don't know whether it was a male or what, how come it was so big. The one in Spain was small, probably five foot, the one in Topanga over six foot. The first night it woke me up. The second night too. I got angry, I started getting annoyed with this stuff. So about the third night, I just fired the covers right off the bed and charged right into it. It kind of popped but there was no sound or anything. If you can imagine a balloon that you can break and it's got water in it. I was really damp. I'll never forget that I had to go take a towel and dry myself off. But the ghost never came back.

Recently, as I studied the transcript of my interview with Jerry, a theory occurred to me about who *this* ghost might have been, the ghost who for a time haunted their house in the Santa Monica Mountains. Jenny had left her previous husband and taken their two small daughters to live with Jerry. But her husband, a highly placed executive, refused to give her a divorce. Soon he became an alcoholic, lost his job, then eventually died of alcoholism. Was he dead, I wondered, by the time the haunting in Topanga began?

Jerry is a friend of mine, so I phoned him and asked him *when* Jenny's first husband died. Around 1968, Jerry replied, before he and his family moved to Topanga. Well then, I asked, mightn't the ghost of Jenny's vindictive ex-husband have been harassing them?

Jerry thought for half a minute and said, "Sure, maybe so." Then he gave me some remarkable news.

I already knew that over the past year, Jerry had broken up with the woman he married after Jenny, and had found a new, more fulfilling partner. Now he told me that Jenny's spirit—out of contact with him for over twenty years—had started visiting both Jerry and his new partner, apparently giving her blessing to his new relationship. Does this sound too sentimental to be true? Not to me, since—as described in Chapter 1—when I started seriously dating my present husband, the spirit of my previous husband made its approving presence known.

Jerry's stories illustrate two different kinds of haunts: those like the ghost in the Balearic Islands that are simply tied to a place, and the personal kind, like Jenny's first husband. An angry or unhappy spirit may hound someone they cared about in life as Jenny's first husband seems to have hassled her. Denise, whose story is told in Chapter 6, was virtually stalked by the ghost of her first husband, a deeply troubled suicide. He disturbed her dreams, called out to her during the day, appeared to their daughter in broad daylight, and woke both Denise's present husband and herself by turning on their bedroom light in the middle of the night.

On the other hand, ghosts tied to a house or a neighborhood may make themselves known fleetingly to strangers who venture onto their turf. When Christina was a young girl, she and her Swedish-born grandmother saw a semi-visible man.

> We were sitting at the dining room table and we looked over to the neighbors' place, about 40 feet away. And we saw this man that was transparent that was walking from their front porch to their back porch. We both looked at him. And I mean there wasn't any type of reflection of any sort, it wasn't something on a window pane or something. Because when he disappeared, it was like that [snapping her fingers]. And my grandmother said, "I saw a man that I could see through." And I said, "Well, I did too." But we didn't know a thing about this man, nothing. And we didn't say anything more about it then. But as I got older, we would talk about it.

Christina's grandmother also told her about a ghost that she'd seen when she was a girl in Sweden.

> Her mother's close friend had died. There was a knock at the door and it was this woman who had died. And my grandmother and her sisters and brothers were just flabbergasted. So they ran for their mother and the mother came to the door but she could not see the woman who was at the door.

When Maxine was newly married, she lived in California in a tiny adobe house that had been built by Mexican laborers who were making adobe brick for huge mansions in the neighborhood. Again and again, she sensed presences in it.

> Before we bought it, it was abandoned for seven years after the woman who owned it died there. When we came to the house, it still had everything just as she left it. Candy next to her bed, Bisquick in the cupboard, everything had been left and it was very interesting. Very fun.
>
> Things would come off shelves, the refrigerator door would open, windows would kind of open. Weird little things like that. The last week that we were in the house before we moved, I woke up in the middle of the night and there right next to me was an older gentleman with a long beard leaning up against the desk looking at me. And of course I freaked out, I gasped—and it was gone. Didn't look like anybody I knew. I woke up my husband. I was in a state.
>
> Somehow in the move a photograph turned up and the picture was like this being that I saw and I nearly came unglued because I hadn't a clue. We were in a tiny house, I hadn't a clue where the heck this picture came from. I don't remember the story behind it but this man had had something to do with the property. A few days later when I'd sort of removed myself, I was tickled by the whole thing. It was kind of a neat experience.

Memories of the Civil War, which exacted over a million casualties, still "haunt" our nation. Little wonder that paranormal haunts continue in its wake. Two of my informants told me about events that hark back to that grisly conflict. Mary-Minn's story recalls the cartoon character, Casper the Friendly Ghost. As a youngster she lived with her grandparents in a haunted house in Iowa.

> I mean, it was written up in the *National Enquirer*, it was on *Good Morning, America*. I was 13 years old and my friends were 15 and 16. We used to go up in the attic and play. My grandparents had at least one Victrola with old-fashioned clay records and there was a lot of old clothing up there including a Civil War uniform with a bullet hole in the chest and we fancied blood in the bullet hole. So we were playing the Victrola and the Civil War uniform started going back and forth on its hanger—there wasn't any wind—and then it just started dancing. It was really scary. We were screaming and yowling. And then we ran down the stairs and the hatboxes which were very neatly stacked on top of each other started rolling down after us. And we were just *screaming*. It was really funny.
>
> Helen used to clean house for my grandmother and she said that she'd be up there with another cleaning lady, Velma, and she'd feel a touch or she'd feel something moving past her and she'd say, "Velma?" and nobody would be there. It was just a known presence, not a malevolent person, a very playful ghost. It played havoc but it never did anything mean. It liked children. According to the people who now own the house, their children have become friends with it. It's not unfriendly, it's just rambunctious, hides socks and stuff.

Anna is a very sensitive woman, several of whose accounts are quoted in earlier chapters. However, when a friend told her about poltergeist-like experiences he had had, where heavy objects seemed to move of their own accord, Anna told her friend she didn't believe in this.

> We were in Virginia and the inn we were eating at had been a Civil War hospital. I no more got this statement out of my mouth, I no more than said "*I* wouldn't want to see a ghost," or "*I* wouldn't want to see something rise off the wall," than right across from me this wreath came out from the wall about two feet straight out and then very slowly dropped. Didn't hurt a thing. And then I said, "That's crazy!" I got up and I said, "I'm gonna use the bathroom." I went in, I sat on the toilet and the toilet seat fell off! I've never! I almost hurt myself. *[Laughing]* I sat down on the toilet and the toilet

seat literally became unconnected to whatever it is. And I caught myself without going all the way to the floor.

Afterwards we asked the waitress about the place. She just stayed and told us story after story. It had been a Civil War hospital. Where we were sitting was the operating room. Outside by that tree I could see was all limbs, you know. And I'm like, who wants to eat a seventy dollar dinner here?

Kevin reported an experience in a motel not unlike Anna's in that restaurant.

A curtain assembly fell off the wall. The whole valence, couple layers of curtains, the whole thing just pulled right out of the wall. And it was stuck in really firmly with 3-inch long plastic things kind of shaped like a diamond, and when you push it in, the diamond squeezes together. If they had torn out of the wall, then you'd have seen it. If the curtains had fallen of their own weight, you would be able to tell. But the whole assembly pulled cleanly out of the wall. The diamond-shaped things pulled totally out of the wall. They had to have been pulled straight out and come down, which is the way a poltergeist kind of thing works. Like, pictures come off the wall straight out and then fall down. I think this was all because of a big frustration going on in my life at the time, after my mother died—but I don't connect it to my mother. I've had lots of stuff like this, psychokinetic things.

Kevin was guessing that he himself was somehow responsible for those curtains falling down. Poltergeist phenomena are often attributed to the psychic influence of emotionally distressed *living* persons—most typically teenagers but sometimes adults as well who share the excitable, high energy level of adolescents. The disturbances they cause in their environment may punish people they dislike or otherwise meet their emotional needs.

The word "poltergeist" comes from German words that mean noisy ghost. It's associated not only with "things that go bump in the night"—raps, rattles, moans, the clink of chains and other trappings of horror movies—but with bricks and rocks clattering on roofs, cupboards flying open, and household objects disappearing and maybe reappearing—often somewhere else—or photogenically flying around. (Except that, typically, when objects take off, observers just spot them out of the corner of their eye.) Often such events recur in a given place, or in connection with a given person, for months or years.

Parapsychologists wrestling with any particular case must decide whether its cause is living or dead. In an article written in 1972, a leading researcher suggested an ingenious screen for distinguishing poltergeist phenomena with a living cause from those brought on by spirit visitors. Among other things he argued that the agent is probably discarnate (no longer endowed with an earthly body) when: a) objects seen flying through the air suddenly change their speed or direction, b) travel more than 15 feet, c) are particularly heavy, d) seem to be carried and deposited gently, e) there is no benefit to the primary perceiver, and f) exorcism or placation convince the agent to stop its troublesome behavior. Judged by these standards, most—but probably not all—of the events reported in this chapter seem to have been caused by discarnate influences.

Both Mary-Minn and Bob, a retired engineer, reported experiences that involved card tables. Here is Mary-Minn's story:

> When I was a kid in Iowa, my friends and I had a seance in which we asked the spirit to talk and the spirit brought up the leg of a folded card table. I mean, it was up against a wall and we had told the spirit to talk. And it moved in an anti-gravitational way. It went up very intentionally.

Here a researcher feels obliged to ask whether the psychic energy of Mary-Minn and her teenage friends was responsible for the movement of this physical object. Maybe so, maybe not. Certainty does not come easy when you study the paranormal. Bob told me this in a written report:

> My parents, my sister and I lived in a two-story house in Sioux Falls, SD. It had a stairway going up the hall wall to a landing where a right angle turn was made onto a hallway. For a while, they stored a card table at the top of the landing. One night it slid down the stairs. The next day, they tried several different ways to knock the

card table over and cause it to slide down the steps. Nothing worked. So they stood the card table back on end in the same place only to hear it slide down the stairs several nights later. They then moved it to a different storage location.

Bob went on to tell a story about a classic haunted house:

> A man hanged himself in the house where my grandparents lived. He was found upstairs. . . . The family dog would run to the door on the first floor that led up the stairs to the second floor, raise his hackles, snarl or growl or bark and then run away very quickly. Pictures that were hung in the upstairs bedrooms always fell down. And thumb locks to the cupboards on the second floor would be closed at night and be found open in the morning. My aunt said you could lie in bed and listen to the thumb locks turning as the metal ground against metal.

A ghost associated with a place threatened Summer very personally. Fortunately this spirit yielded to a ritual of placation.

> When Tom and I first moved in together, we were living in a little trailer on one of the last farms in Bolinas, [*in Northern California*]. Jerry Garcia lived there and Starship had a house there. Lots of musicians. Beautiful.
>
> Our second night in the trailer we made love and went to sleep and I had a dream. I dreamt that I was in a beautiful little vacation house. I was in the living room, standing right in front of the sofa and I saw a mist. And it became like a puff of smoke and then it became a head, and then shoulders started to form, and as it started to form it started towards me. And it was a *male* spirit. I knew that much. And just as it got to me, the hands and the torso were formed. It took me by the shoulders and started to push me gently but firmly down on the sofa. And it had very much of a sexual feeling to it and I woke up in terror. Woke Tom up and told him about it. And the next day we talked to the family whose land we were on.
>
> The old man's name was Leo. Leo's older brother had lived in that trailer and had died of a heart attack in that trailer. Tom had lived there for a while and never had any experiences. So we asked them and they told us about their wonderful older brother and uncle and his name was Incensio and they called him Incense. We didn't

tell them why we were asking. I always thought we woke his spirit up making love or something. Kinda turned him on!

It scared me a little. I didn't want to make it with Incensio, so Tom and I said well, we'll do a little exorcism. So that evening we just sat down on the floor. We lit a candle and we burned some incense and we drank a little wine and we said, "Incense, thank you for letting us stay in your place. We're just here for a while to save money so we can buy land so we can have our farm and have our family too. Thank you for letting us live on your wonderful farm, and please may we stay here until after the harvest. We didn't mean to disturb you or anything, and we ask that you not frighten us. And we don't want to frighten you." We blew the candle out and went to bed and that was that. Never had any other bad feelings.

The most frightening ghost experience may well be possession—sensing that the spirit of a dead being has taken over your body and your will. In the movies, our heroine is taken over by a demon. None of my informants was as accursed as all that. Nonetheless, several reported sensing another's spirit within them. One exhibited so much entanglement with her late husband that two local psychics offered to attempt exorcisms and she—in character—complied.

Doris is a brilliant woman in her thirties whom I interviewed a few years after she was widowed. She holds graduate degrees in two different demanding fields. But from earliest childhood she was sexually abused by an alcoholic uncle who lived nearby. This continuing experience left her "badly crushed." It blurred her sense of who she was and made it virtually impossible for her to express anger, particularly since her older sister made her promise never to tell her parents about her uncle's assaults on her "because the adults already had too many problems and it would worry them. It was a heavy duty, I'm still recovering. I'm still finding ways to be present and involved rather than masked and methodical and functional through patterned learning."

In her mid-twenties, she met and married Julian, a successful man twice her age who was highly opinionated and outspoken. She willingly let him direct her life. He inculcated his ideas and point of view in her and encouraged her to go to graduate school. After he died seven years later, she sensed that he was still influencing her choices and expressing himself through her speech.

> A lot of that time *[the first two months after his death]* he was riding my shoulder, sitting right on me. And he was laughing. People would come over and we'd let 'em have it, right? Only it was Julian talking a lot of the time.
>
> He was talking through me. I mean, I had become so malleable to him. He came and spoke through me and a lot of the time I don't know what condition I might have been in. I think I had a little bit of alcohol now and then. He was quite the drunk but I tended to do very little. I was in school. I was so distraught, I was pretty devastated. And he would come. I was pretty much down to a very small bit of self and Julian was still there.
>
> I don't know why he was around so much except that I don't think he was done and I think I was holding him back from going because I'd gotten so wrapped up in him. But there's a sort of strange dreadfulness about keeping a person around who's dead. I am still just building myself up to have an existence.
>
> One night about a year after he died, I was living in the country in an area where there were several households on a piece of property. One fellow had a New Year's party that was very gentle and sweet. I went outside and I was looking up at a beautiful clear sky, no moon I remember. So the stars were very bright in the middle of winter and Orion was there and Julian was overlaid on Orion and talking to me. And at that point was a real comfort. I mean, it was like he was that far away now. It was like he was *other,* he wasn't inside me.

Nonetheless, when Doris continued to feel Julian's presence exerting an untamable, often raucous influence over her daily life, she let others in her spiritual community try to send him away.

> There were two events, sort of soul retrieval things, where people were trying to get him out of me. The first one found a strong presence of Julian and that was a negative thing from her perspective. I let her do what she could and would. I did the visualizations and an animal spirit came to help pull him out of me. And then him giving me back myself and me giving him back himself. And seeing

him go, moving away. And then a big black wall slammed down and I couldn't tell what happened after that. It was like, "No, stay out of here, this is not your business." Still I think it probably lightened the bond.

The second time was with another woman who was a healer and a teacher. It was a process with drumming and chanting and there were students. And she was calling in the spirits and she was telling me what to do. Put those ones out, pull up this shell. I don't remember all the details. But the part about Julian was very easy. There was no resistance. And there were two friendly spirits there to be with him.

By the time I interviewed Doris, she no longer felt controlled by Julian. Still he returned to her occasionally.

When he comes and is with me, he usually sits sort of between my neck and my right shoulder, [*motioning*] on the back of my shoulder on the top of my back. Like a tiny elf, eight, ten inches high that embodies the whole big Julian. He's there and I can be a puppet if I decide I want to. And he's wanting me to. A puppet isn't quite it. It's more like my body becomes his body and he can use it. For his own expressions and things.

It happens maybe every couple of months. I tend to not allow it full strength ever. And I check the person I'm talking with to see if I really want to do Julian on 'em. How long? I rest with it, I dream with it for maybe 15 minutes or an hour. Or half a day if it's not very strong.

Is Doris's experience truly possession? Or does it combine love and grief and the need of a damaged person to excuse her own increasingly bold behavior by attributing it to the spirit of her late husband? Often we gradually acquire personality traits that we admired in those we loved. For instance, when I was married to Paul, I was more introverted and shy than I am now. After his death, I gradually took on some of his more gregarious style. But I've never attributed this change in my behavior to possession.

On the other hand, it's not unusual in an after-death communication for the perceiver to sense another's spirit taking over.

Sometimes this is a pleasant feeling. Thus, as reported in Chapter 2, John sensed his friend and mentor, Harper, at the time of Harper's death. "I was just filled with the sense of him. It was a feeling of intense euphoria, like he was within me or we were one. I was overwhelmed by his presence and it was all positive."

The day that the father of Carol's longtime partner died, he seemed to take her over and control her behavior.

> I met Irv in 1980 when I was 23. He and I became really good buddies, he took me out fishing. I'll never say that Irv was a surrogate dad but we were definitely close and he also was very supportive of me through the whole ending of my relationship with his son—and after. He died in Canada in 1993. That morning I was in Los Angeles with my mom and we were walking along the beach just before I was supposed to get on the plane to go back to Victoria, B.C. where I was living. My mom is a social worker trained in hypnotherapy and she wanted to do some hypnosis with me. I started getting increasingly cantankerous and just very pissy—and cantankerous is definitely a word that could be used to describe Irv.
>
> It got very intense. I finally freaked out on my mom and I said, "You know what? I can't *do* this. We have to *stop* it, just *stop* it. . . ." And my mom was going like, "*What* is your *problem?* Jeeze, you're cantankerous!" I don't know if she used that word but certainly something very similar. I got very bitchy. I didn't arrive back in Victoria until that evening around 8 or 9 at night. I got back to a message that Irv had died that morning. He died right when that whole thing happened on the beach.

Elise is a natural medium. When she and her professor husband were visiting the battlefield at Gettysburg, she was possessed by the spirit of someone who was wounded there 130 years before. Strange as that experience was, ultimately she felt enriched by it.

> We're driving. We get to this area that's called Big Round Top. There's Little Round Top and Big Round Top, two sites of the battle. It's in the morning. I am *not* tired, I'd had plenty of sleep. But as we pulled into the park I felt like somebody had given me a tranquilizer and put me under. I could not stay awake. I went sound asleep and I was like fighting it. But I went to sleep within that ten minutes. I

woke up when he parked the car. As we walked across the street into this area of Little Round Top, I said "Greg, I don't feel like myself." All of a sudden, here comes the professor. You know, the scientist. He pulls out a pad of paper and a pencil and starts asking me questions. I've gotten used to it now, okay? He starts asking me questions and writing down answers—which is a good thing because when something like this happens I wouldn't remember it if not for him. It'd be like a dream. It's like my mind went to a theta or a delta state and I would not have remembered it.

I started by saying, "I keep wanting to talk to Sarah, I've got to talk to Sarah." He wanted to know who Sarah was and I said, "I've got to write a letter to Sarah." Pretty soon I had some other symptoms—I'm limping. I was able to point to where I felt my legs were hurt—bottom of one leg and the thigh on the other—and I'm looking at him and saying, "This is nuts." I'm walking with this rolling gait and I'm telling him about the amount of pain I have and I point exactly and he writes down the places.

He came over behind me and he goes, "Oh, my gosh." Behind me was hot as Hades. His hand was out two or three feet from me and he felt all this heat behind me. Then I started to talk. I was comparing what it looked like that day to what it had been like in 1863 on that Fourth of July weekend this person had been there. I was talking about being cooler, I was talking about how quiet it was. I could look down and see what had been there such as pools of blood on the rocks and so on. At the same time I could see reality. It was like one was superimposed over the other. I could hear all the sound that was there before and could realize how quiet it was now. The person who was with me was making these comparisons. And then he started philosophizing.

I had the most unusual experience of my life. I had never understood war or killing. I had understood patriotism but I had never understood killing. And this man starts talking about Alexander the Great, which I know nothing about. He starts talking about a cause and he was eloquent. And all of a sudden, I had the experience of understanding and reframing that whole battle into something that was so honorable. I truly understood the word "honor." I could truly understand why they did that, I could understand the man's *pride* in what they'd done.

Well, my husband called a fellow who's written books about Gettysburg. He asked if he'd heard of any such thing. And it turned out that this fellow had been doing research on a man named Joshua Chamberlain who was injured in precisely the same spots on his legs that I was pointing to. By the way, when I left that place, I walked just regular and felt just fine. I wasn't sleepy.

This Joshua Chamberlain, his mother was Sarah and his sister was Sarah. He didn't die at Gettysburg. He went on to become president of Bowdoin College and governor of Maine. He was a philosophy professor before he went into the Civil War. His family tried to keep him out of it by having him go to Europe—but he believed he had to fight. He lived into his nineties. He just came in to use my eyes and my senses. It was like he stopped in to take a look after 130 years. There was that feeling of honor, there was this pride in his men. There were all these feelings that I would never have understood if I had not been the channel or the vehicle.

15

What's So Different About Paranormal Dreams?

AFTER-DEATH COMMUNICATION can come via many routes: the five senses, symbolic events, and telepathy, among others. One of the most puzzling of these routes is dreams. Ordinarily we think of dreams as fantasies which, however symbolic, tend to jumble together all kinds of misleading clues. Though I myself have had numerous contact experiences, I've generally sensed them via concrete indications during my waking hours—flashing lights, moving objects and the like. So I asked my dream-perceivers what made their paranormal dreams different. What alerted the dreamer to their significance?

Of course, when a dream communicates something verifiable that the dreamer never knew before, its significance can't be questioned. In three of the death coincidences described in Chapter 2, women learned through dreams that other women they'd been close to had just died and now were happy. Similarly, there are many cases in the literature of the paranormal where a person learns through a dream where to locate a lost object. A friend of mine told me that just this had happened in her family. Her aunt had a dream in which her dead grandfather told her where she could find some valuable jewelry. Dreams like this impress us with their importance because they jibe with information that comes to the dreamer later. But even when an ADC dream isn't followed by a confirming revelation, something about it tends to trigger an intense response.

Virtually all my informants agreed that, unlike the run-of-the-mill variety which generally fade from memory as soon as you wake, their contact dreams stayed with them, often for years, often in remarkable detail. And sometimes when they woke, they discovered other signs that their contact had been real. After Beverly lost her husband, she went into a period of deep grief and shut herself off from the world. Here's how she described a dream she had two years after the death of her husband and three years before our interview.

> I was walking and there were stores on each side of a cobblestone walkway and there were fountains in the middle and I went to walk into this one store and my husband just stepped out in the doorway. And he hugged me and he said, 'Let's go walk,' so we walked to the fountain and he said, 'You have to go on with your life. You can't *do* this anymore.' He says, 'I'm okay but *you* have to get on with your life'.... So anyway we continued to talk at the fountain, then he gave me a hug and left. Now, when I woke up I could smell—I hadn't had any of his stuff around for the last couple of years—but I could smell all over my body Royal Copenhagen *[her husband's cologne]* so I knew we had met somewhere. Although it appeared to be in the physical realm, I knew it wasn't. I knew I was *with him.*

A few years before I interviewed Melissa, the man she considered her soulmate died. Melissa's description recalls many near-death experience accounts which stress the intensity and beauty of a rustic scene.

> I've had two very vivid dreams where he's come and been clear as day. I knew he was dead in my dream but he was coming to tell me that he loved me very much and in one of them, that things were gonna be okay, I would be happy again, and he wanted me to be happy and not be sad that he was dead and it was so *clear.* We were by this river in a deep woods with tall trees which we both loved dearly—we both used to hike a lot. And he just came to me on the bank of the river and he had like a white tee shirt on and jeans. And

it was as *clear,* just as clear as if he had been alive, and he was very healthy. Everything was so vivid—the colors of the trees, the smells of the woods, the water in the river.

Dreams like this make an enduring mark on their perceivers. Here's how they were described by three of my informants.

It's like you're in the physical realm. I dream all the time but the minute I wake up I never remember my dream. I mean, they just pass and if I could remember little portions of them I can never put them all together and I can't really remember details. In these dreams I can remember details. I can visually see them. And I can recall the feeling of the touch when [my late husband] put his arms around me. And each time after I woke up, I felt a glorious, deep sense of peace.

These are dreams that I remembered as opposed to just, you know, not remembering. They had an impact on me, a deeper impact on me. So whether they're actual experiences or whether they were just dream experiences I couldn't say. Except that they had a lasting impact on me.

The experiences are extremely intense. I mean, they're just as though the person is right there and it's happening. I mean it's very very intense. And very wonderful when they happen, I might add. There's never been a negative effect from it. I've never had an experience of impending doom or warning or anything. Always been a very positive kind of thing.

Denise felt hounded by her late ex-husband. Though her dreams of him were negative, they were just as intense.

I guess it's kind of a cliché but I'd wake up feeling that they were so real. That everything with him in it was so real. Some other dreams could feel real, but every one with him was so real that I woke up feeling like I was just in his world or something. Like we came and met in a different area. I woke up just *knowing.* The brain isn't thinking, it's the intuition, and I'd wake up knowing that was him coming to me.

After Yona's brother-in-law died of cancer, he came to her in a dream. Peter, a teacher, had a cheerfully inquiring mind.

> I hardly ever remember dreams. That was interesting. This dream was about seeing Pete outside of their house, in the pickup truck. And I was like, "Pete, what are you doing here!" *[Laughs]* I knew he was dead. And he said, "Oh, I've been going around doing this and that." I said, "Pete, I've been wanting to talk to you because if you're on the other side, there are all these people that you could ask some pretty amazing questions." And he said, "Oh, I've been doing that." He had a fanny pack and he had his notes and that was just like him. It was like, wow! And there was something about that he was invisible to some people because some kids knew he was there and some kids wouldn't. It was very realistic for me.
>
> I'm not sure of my beliefs, one way or the other, but it made total sense that this guy was on the other side. He was limitless and he was checking this and that out. And he was just like his usual self.

Two people mentioned dreams with a strikingly golden look. First, from Marti:

> I generally dream in black and white but the dreams where I believe he made contact were like a sepia photo except that, instead of that pinkish brown, it was gold, yellowy gold.

After Dorothy lost her daughter Amy, a family friend told her about a dream he had which he didn't understand at the time. It came to him after Amy had been hospitalized with brain injuries from a car accident.

> He described it vividly. It was about 5:30 a.m. *[around the time when Amy's condition worsened; that evening she died.]* He saw this beautiful light—clear, golden, vivid colors. Amy was there. Her sister was a few paces behind her right shoulder. He tried to step around Amy to get to her sister but Amy stepped in front to say, "Tell my family I love them." She tried to say more. Her mouth moved but he heard no sound. Two days later, he picked up the local newspaper, saw a photo of Amy, and wondered what good event she'd been

involved in. The article was her obituary. That was how he first learned of her death.

Other informants told of having ADCs which interrupted more run-of-the-mill dreams. On several occasions while sleeping, Jan has received paranormal messages for others.

> I have wonderful dreams. I describe them as being Cecil B. deMille productions. I remember and see details in my dreams but quite often I don't know anyone in them. As a young girl, I used to dream a lot that I got married but the person that I married never had a face. It was just kind of grayed out.
>
> So I dream wonderful, detailed dreams but very seldom do I ever know *anybody* in the dream. It's an event that's happening to me, an experience that's going on, a place where I am. When these people with messages came to me, it was as though they came into an *existing* dream to kind of take a little break. They stopped the motion as if to say I'm gonna tell you something. And then disappeared out of the dream. It's so different when these people come to me.

Maxine has often sensed contact with her beloved grandmother since she died.

> She would come to me and say, "Everything is fine. Just don't worry, I'm here." They were incredibly comforting, really comforting dreams. She would pop in. The dreams I have about her—it's usually once a year—they always come at a time when I'm floundering or needing something, a dose of something. And she'll just show up, she'll just be there. And she'll smile in her funny little way. And she'll shake her finger at me in a loving, endearing sort of way. And that's really all I need.
>
> A few months ago she just appeared out of nowhere. The dream had nothing to do with anything and here she stepped in—and yet the next morning it was so obviously right that she came at that point.

Seventeen years before I interviewed Vicki, her infant daughter—at that time, an only child—died of crib death. Since Vicki had gone through the anguish of a miscarriage before the birth of her daughter, she felt terrified of trying to have another child. Then what she calls a dream-vision changed her mind.

> Within a month after April died, I had trouble sleeping. I'd get up in the middle of the night. My husband would be sleeping and I'd listen to every breath he took because of the fear of losing him. I mean, it was an irrational kind of thing. I would read the Bible trying to find answers. I wanted to know why, why did this seemingly perfectly healthy baby forget to breathe? Now I figure probably I'll never have any answers.
>
> I've never remembered dreams unless it was like a nightmare and then I wake up and maybe remember fragments, but not very much. But this thing was . . . I hesitate to call it a dream because I don't remember dreams so it's like a dream vision kind of thing. But I was in bed and April came back to me and my mom [*who was still alive*] was there too. And she was holding April and she handed her to me for just a minute and I turned to my mom and I said, "See, she *is* in a good place, she really is in a good place," and then I went to hand her to my mom and April just vanished and at that point I was alert. And I just laid there for hours just thinking *what just happened?* And I've never, never since had anything that powerful.

This dream vision gave Vicki the courage to risk getting pregnant again. When I interviewed her she was a skilled technician in an educational program and the proud mother of two healthy children.

16

Who Becomes a Sensitive?

A BRIEF VISION CHANGED VICKI'S LIFE FOREVER, and for the better. Nonetheless in our society, folks who describe psi experiences they've had, put themselves at risk of ridicule or worse. An intimidating gulf yawns between the believers and the non-believers, between those who on occasion gain knowledge via psychic routes and everybody else.

Typically, people who sense contact with the dead have a knack for other kinds of clairvoyance as well. For instance, they're likely to get upset and somehow know when someone dear to them is in an accident. Something like this happened to Vicki when she was still in high school. She was out on a date with her husband-to-be when she suddenly sensed that she had to hurry home. Soon she discovered that her brother had frolicked into the woods with friends and had rolled his pickup down an embankment. Even though he wasn't seriously injured, Vicki picked up some paranormal hint that he was in danger.

Women and men who are even more psychic than Vicki may be able to find things that others have mislaid, or may feel prompted to give a message to a friend that someone *that* person cares about will need an operation or soon will come on a visit. Several of the people I interviewed were natural mediums. How, I wondered, did they get their extraordinary powers?

It's not that sensitivity to the paranormal is rare. It isn't. As Chapter 1 documents, the majority of the world's widows and almost as large a percentage of widowers sense some sort of after-death contact with their lost partners soon after bereavement. As the novelist Willa Cather wrote, "Where there is great love there are always miracles." And as this whole book demonstrates, ADCs are hardly limited to people who have lost their partners.

Almost a third of Americans polled by CBS News in 1998 said they believed that "some people have the ability to communicate with spirits or with people that have died." An earlier poll showed 27% of Americans reporting that, on at least one occasion, they themselves had sensed contact with someone who had died. Clairvoyance, sensing events happening at a great distance, was reported by 24% while, when asked about sensing a telepathic connection with a living person, positive responses rose to a striking 58%.

Looking at data from other countries, (Table 1) we find widely varying numbers that show little pattern according to region. Even within a given country, scores may be high for one experience and low for another. Thus, in Iceland, a whopping 41% reported contact with the dead and 33% reported telepathy, but only 7% reported clairvoyance. The highest overall scores came from Italy, where 33% had sensed contact with the dead, and telepathy and clairvoyance each drew responses of 38%. At least 23% of Britons, West Germans and French reported contact with the dead experiences. And in most Western European nations, telepathy was reported by at least a quarter of the population. Clearly, a great many people are occasionally sensitive to at least some form of psi. But what makes some people far more psychic than others?

When I planned my study, I hoped to uncover some of the factors that tend to create sensitives. In my questionnaire, I didn't just ask about psi experiences my informants might have had. I also asked about their childhood training and adult beliefs regarding both traditional religion and the supernatural or paranormal—whichever word felt most comfortable to the interviewee. I was hoping to learn: Did being brought up in a traditional faith make you more or less likely to have ADCs? And how about people who'd been brought up to believe in a spirit world that could interact with the living on earth?

Table 1.
Percentage of persons in the Human Values Survey
reporting the following experiences:

	Telepathy	Clairvoyance	Contact with the Dead
Great Britain	36	14	26
Northern Ireland	24	11	12
Rep. of Ireland	19	11	16
West Germany	35	15	26
Holland	27	12	11
Belgium	18	12	16
France	34	24	23
Italy	38	38	33
Spain	20	13	16
Malta	28	18	19
Denmark	14	11	9
Sweden	23	7	14
Finland	35	15	15
Norway	18	7	9
Iceland	33	7	41
Total for Western Europe	32	20	23
U.S.A.	58	24	27

Source: E. Haraldsson. (October 1985) "Representative national surveys of psychic phenomena." *Journal of the Society for Psychical Research, 53, 801, 147.*

It soon became clear that past religious training had little to do with receptivity to psi. People who had been raised to be atheists or devout, Catholic, Protestant or Jewish, seemed equally likely to show psychic tendencies. But psychic tendencies themselves seemed to run in families. Several of my informants told me that their mother was psychic. If not mom, then somebody else in the family. Aunt Jane told fortunes with cards. Or when grandma lived on a farm, she always knew what was happening in town even though they didn't have a phone. The day that Michael almost died in a fire in Denmark, his brother felt so alarmed that he started phoning him every half hour from the United States until at last he reached him. And more than once I heard of mothers who sensed their daughters' labor pains.

Charles is a winning young man whom I know to be responsible and honest. He has a twin brother and, for generations, twins have abounded in his family. "On both sides," he told me, "I have cousins and uncles and aunts that are all twins." Folklore and systematic research agree that twins often sense from afar what's happening to their birth mates so it's likely that for generations Charles's forebears have had lots of experience with ESP. What's more, Charles's mother comes from a long line of women psychics. So I wasn't quite so astonished as I might have been when he told me stories about his mother that recalled the occasional science fiction film.

> Mom has had many many experiences on her own. When my grandfather was dying, they put him in the hospital. Then on the day he died, my mother was pacing outside of his bedroom. She swears she heard music, she heard bells and harps. It scared her. She walked into my grandpa's room and about ten minutes later, he flat-lined.
>
> She says she can create electricity where there is no electricity. When she was six or seven years old, it had just gotten dark and my grandma was making dinner in the kitchen, so she told my mom to go out to the garage and grab a bag of potatoes. The garage had just been built four or five months previously. It had outlets and light fixtures but there was no power that had ever been connected. They hadn't put the line across and it was pretty empty. So my mom went out there and flipped on the light switch and the light came on in the garage. My grandma kind of looked out there and thought to herself, "Now what in the world? Did she grab a lantern? What's going on?" And she walked out there and there was light coming out of the light socket! No light bulb and no power—but there was light!
>
> And my mother started a fire once when they went camping and they ran out of matches. She stood there, just stood over the wood, frustrated, just looking at it and looking at it and there it was! It just started smoking down at the bottom. She says she's had endless examples of these things.
>
> My mother didn't tell me these stories till I was 21 years old and I'd moved away—then moved back in. I was just sitting there having

dinner with her. She said, "Did you know I'm a freak?" And I looked at her and said, "What do you mean, you're a freak?" And she's like, "Oh, never mind. I'll tell you someday." Then about three months later, she's like, "Sit down. I want to tell you some stories."

Little wonder that for years Charles's mother didn't dare confide in her son. In an earlier age, she'd have been burned as a witch for sure! From a parapsychologist's point of view, she's not just psychic, she's endowed with unusual—but not unheard of—telekinetic powers. In the old Soviet Union, scientific research was done with men and women who, among other things, could make freestanding light bulbs glow. On TV, I've seen film footage that testifies to this. When the Soviet's most powerful telekinetic medium, Ninel Kulagina, was checked under laboratory conditions, she appeared to draw electrical energy from around her into her body, then discharge it at a target object to make it move. Kulagina could move objects as heavy as a pound without touching them—but the effort drained her of energy. Sometimes rushes of energy afterwards into her depleted body left burn marks on her skin and set her clothes on fire.

Charles's stories about his mother's remarkable experiences seemed more plausible because she came from a long line of psychic women and men. As children, many were probably encouraged to gain information psychically. Sociologist Charles Emmons has described this process. "One third-generation spirit medium said that when she told her mother that there was a man standing in the corner, her mother asked, 'What's his name?' . . . Another medium reports that her grandmother used to play psychic games with her (e.g., hide a key and say, 'Become the key, then see where you are.')"

Recently, hard evidence that psi often runs in families has come from the study of second sight. "Second sight" is a catchall label for a number of related psychic gifts. It can cover prophetic visions of happy events like marriages or, more often, calamities like deaths or accidents. Sometimes people with second sight have a waking vision of a person who at that moment is dying elsewhere—in other words, they experience a death coincidence.

Second sight is known to be particularly common in the Scottish Highlands and Western Isles. Dr. Shari Cohn, a young American researcher who lives and works in Scotland, has been studying it for some time.

In the early 1990s, Cohn distributed a lengthy questionnaire to Scots and people of Scottish ancestry living abroad, most of whom had experienced psi; she received 208 completed responses. The questionnaire covered not only various kinds of psychic experiences but family patterns of psi receptivity. It's probably not surprising that almost 10% of those who returned her questionnaire were twins—though only 1 in 40 of the general population is a twin. Many of those who *weren't* twins reported that they had twins in their family. Later in the decade, Cohn analyzed 130 family histories and using standard methods from genetics determined that there was a strong tendency for second sight to run in families.

Dr. Cohn found that, just as with ADCs, women are more likely to have second sight than men; they also have more psi experiences of other sorts than men. Families, she reports, "regarded second sight as being both a spiritual and physical phenomenon. . . . There was a deep belief in fate, that what was seen would happen and that one could generally not intervene. . . . Also . . . that when a person dies, some part of them, a soul, continues. In some families with second sight, it was . . . believed to be a hereditary 'gift.' In other families, the subject was taboo. Yet despite this, it still ran in these families."

My own research revealed that, even when informants didn't come from families where anyone admitted to having sensed psi, as children many had been close to people who talked and read about the paranormal. One woman had attended a Waldorf School devoted to the occult ideas of Rudolf Steiner, one man's father was fascinated by Edgar Cayce, another's was an amateur magician who often used his young son as a willing hypnotic subject. Almost a third of my interviewees reported that, as kids, they had often heard positive things about the paranormal. It seems clear that early exposure to belief in psi is related to psi sensitivity. But what, I wondered, about the other two thirds of my interviewees—most of whom were raised to deeply mistrust any such thing?

Early in my research I stumbled onto some unexpected patterns. For many of those I interviewed, I guess I was the first person they'd ever spoken to who both admitted to having had paranormal experiences and who wanted noncritically to hear their stories. People poured out to me the most amazing confidences. I'll always be grateful to them—and I sincerely hope that they'll never have cause to regret their trust in me.

By the time I'd interviewed my first fifteen or so informants, something odd had struck me. Four or five had mentioned having alcoholic parents. This although, according to the National Council on Alcoholism and Drug Dependence, only about 7% of the adult American population has serious problems with drinking, and no major decline in alcoholism had occurred since these perceivers were children.

So I added a deliberately vague inquiry to my questionnaire: "Would you say that your childhood was generally pleasant or was it difficult?" I tried to get back to those whom I'd already interviewed who hadn't covered this issue in their earlier responses. And I asked this question of all my later informants. If the answer was "generally pleasant," I didn't pursue it further. (Those too embarrassed to discuss whatever anguish they might have suffered as kids were spared such pain—so my numbers on such problems are probably an undercount.) But if the answer was "difficult" or "both pleasant and difficult," I asked for details.

Over a third of the people for whom I collected these data reported having one or two alcoholic parents. Others reported that an alcoholic relative, an uncle or grandfather, was present in the household. One woman's mother was addicted, instead, to prescription opiates. When this woman was three, her mother smothered her. Only the intervention of a doctor who lived across the street brought her back to life.

Many adult children of alcoholics reported suffering frequent beatings or seeing others in their family frequently beaten. Even where there wasn't significant physical or sexual abuse, there was likely to be massive neglect and other problems. The daughter of an alcoholic mother recalled that when she and her sister came home from school, they never knew whether they'd find her passed out on the kitchen floor. The son of two drunkards said that, though there was no physical abuse in his home, there were lots of battles between his parents about child rearing and paying bills. "All kinds of strange things that kids shouldn't have to deal with, we had to deal with on a regular basis. It's sort of the Jekyll and Hyde story. You become ultra-sensitive in order to judge the current state of affairs with one or the other parent. The drunker they are, the more Mr. Hyde they are."

Soon another "difficult" pattern emerged in the early life of sensitives. Almost a third—primarily *not* from alcoholic homes— reported that they'd come from authoritarian homes where instant, total obedience was demanded, or that they had unloving parents with quick, fiery tempers which they often unleashed on their children. Here are some of their memories of childhood:

> Unthinking obedience was demanded. We were not allowed to fight, we were not allowed to say no, we had to jump when we were spoken to. I'm the only one that was never beaten with a strap. The others [her older siblings] all got it.

> My father was very controlling, strong on discipline and not very loving.

> My mother was real psychotic. She never knew whether she wanted to love me or hate me or kill me, so most of my childhood she just beat me up a lot.

> My father [a minister] was the product of an alcoholic father. He never drank but he was a dry drunk so he used to beat the living daylights out of us and was also very verbally abusive—and then he'd get up in the pulpit and preach love.

The people who reported such backgrounds tended to do so calmly, reflectively, though often with an edge of bitterness. Somehow they had managed to grow beyond their early pain. These were survivors, made strong by the trauma of their childhoods. A growing body of scientific evidence confirms that this can happen. As psychiatrists Eitan Schwarz and Bruce Perry put it in a 1994 article, "consistent daily stress can result in more adaptive later behavior and resiliency."

Some of the most sensitive of my interviewees—women and men who had had numerous ADCs and were clairvoyant in other ways as well—had experienced both these kinds of stress as children: alcoholism in the home plus the oppressive syndrome that I've labeled authoritarian/angry/abusive (an A/A/A upbringing.) Here's how one man, a successful writer and educator, described his childhood:

It was a nightmare. Both my parents were alcoholics. They split up after four years of marriage. My father took my older brother and moved across the continent. For a while my mother kept me. Then I remember, I'm in the bathtub and I'm saying, "I want my daddy," and she holds my head under water. Damned near drowned me. She didn't want me, I was too much of a nuisance, so she let me go.

I was in jail four times when I was a kid. Had probably the poorest family in the area. My father was the town drunk, we had no mother. We lived in a three room shack in the forest. In the summer, my brother and I had fish to eat out of the stream that ran by the back door. We had blueberries, blackberries and raspberries to eat and we had a pit some distance away where I could go and hit frogs on the head. That was our summer fare many times. [Wry laughter] But in the wintertime in New England it gets very cold. We would hike three miles through the forest to where there was a roadhouse and raid their garbage cans, my brother and I.

Did my father beat me? My dad? Oh, oh, incredible. It was all he knew. But, God bless him, he's the only thing we had. He didn't care if I beat up people. If I went to jail, that didn't seem to bother him. But if I missed school. . . . I ditched school one day and I thought well, I'll go home and I'll sit in the chair, you know. I won't get up and then he won't hit me. Well he came in and picked up the chair with me in it. [Laughing] And he hit me. That's the kind of life we had.

I have yet to locate any other research directly connecting alcoholism in the home or an A/A/A upbringing to paranormal awareness but many have noted a connection between childhood trauma and mediumistic powers. Brad Steiger, who for decades has interviewed mediums and other psychically gifted individuals, reports that "nearly every medium has undergone a series of personal crises in his childhood or youth." He cites an observation by Dr. Gardner Murphy, former president of the American Psychological Association, that "severe illness, things that are biologically or in a broad sense personal crises—disrupting, alerting situations" may lead to heightened psychic awareness. Nonetheless, Steiger notes that most mediums—few of whom earn their living as psychics—are well-adjusted, enthusiastic extroverts of at least average intelligence. They work at a wide range of occupations.

In 1973, a sociological study of 1,460 Americans measured both the frequency of their psychic experiences and significant aspects of their childhood homes. Each was asked: Were your mother and father close to each other? Were you close to your mother? Close to your father? How strict was each of your parents with you? In findings that recalled Steiger's, adult psychics turned out to be a fairly happy, healthy lot. "For those who are highest on the Psi Scale, their experiences seem to correlate with both positive life satisfaction now and anticipations of high life satisfactions five years from now.... [*Perhaps because their adult lives are so much more pleasant than their childhoods were.*] Psychics are ... better educated, no more religious in the conventional sense of the word, and yet more confident of their religious beliefs than the general population." Where childhood stress was concerned, this study found that:

- Though psychics were only slightly more likely to remember tensions in their family's relationships, those who had had frequent psychic experiences, reported higher levels of family tension.

- The relationship between psi and family tension seemed particularly strong for men.

- In general, frequent psi experience seemed to be "caused," at least in part, by growing up in a tense family. This seemed to be most true for the better educated, males, whites, Protestants, and the old.

In the 1980s and early 1990s, several psychologists noticed that people who had endured severe stress in childhood were particularly likely to report having psychic experiences. Since most of them, faithful to the culture's taboo against the paranormal, doubted that there was any *real basis* for such experiences, these researchers concluded that suffering kids developed a tendency to fantasize. In time this might lead them to believe in the paranormal and, ultimately, to imagine psi events. But then the British psychologist Tony Lawrence, using a series of statistical tests, showed that a stronger link existed between trauma and psychic experience than between trauma and fantasy. "You have this direct link from childhood trauma to paranormal experience.... And you don't necessarily need to be a good fantasizer to get that paranormal experience coming in.... Even people with low levels of childhood fantasy could still experience the paranormal because they have trauma in their lives."

Reading Lawrence's papers, I started realizing the many forms that childhood trauma might take. Kids could be scarred not just by melodramatic problems like persistent neglect or sexual and physical abuse, but by deaths in the family, parental divorce, personal illness or repeated moves from one town to another. When I started probing for these kinds of problems in my interviews, I found that several who otherwise came from happy homes, had been psychologically battered by frequent uprootings in their early years. Or by being the son or daughter of a school principal or a clergyman and so always expected to be a model child.

Several of my most sensitive informants reported that, as kids, they'd had both a cheerful introduction to psi and lots of family trauma. One warm, achieving woman who has had loads of ADCs told her story this way:

> My uncle and my grandmother lived together not far from me. They used to read [books about the paranormal] when I was really little so I always had kind of a connection to that. I came from a really dysfunctional family. My mother and my dad and then my stepdad. My dad was an alcoholic, my mother wasn't. I don't know about my stepdad but he had just an incredibly fiery temper. And my mother kind of egged people on, like she was an instigator of confusion.

When my mother and my stepdad would be fighting, they would fight with knives and blood. I mean, they got serious. I used to sit outside beside a fish pool we had and just kind of look at the stars— or sit in the rain, if that was what was happening—and pretend like I was adopted. Being the only child, I had no one other than the animals to buffer—except for my grandmother and my uncle.

It seems clear that coming from a background where psi is accepted, increases your chances of having psi powers. Sadly enough, it would also seem that the child who lives in habitual fear of verbal, physical or sexual abuse, of disruptive and chaotic acts by adults, is especially likely to grow into a sensitive. The first ten years of life are pivotal.

Recent findings about how the human brain develops may help explain much about receptivity to psi. Neurologists now believe that, during a baby's first years, its brain "produces trillions more connections between neurons than it can possibly use. Then [starting around the age of 10 or earlier] . . . the brain eliminates connections, or synapses, that are seldom or never used." This process is related to many skills which are best acquired when you're very young. So, for instance, it's almost impossible to learn to speak a language without a foreign accent unless you start before the age of ten. And the great majority of people with absolute pitch—the ability to identify the tone they hear as C, for example, or E or F sharp—started studying music when they were no older than four or five. It's virtually impossible to acquire absolute pitch—also called perfect pitch—as an adult.

It's easy to speculate that early positive exposure to the paranormal might alert a child to its existence and encourage her to pay attention to non-physical signals. It's trickier to explain why *trauma* might sensitize the developing mind to psi. Maybe, as suggested above, the kid who must constantly navigate treacherous waters becomes "ultra-sensitive in order to judge the current state of affairs."

Some recent work by neurobiologists suggests a more subtle chain of events. Children who are traumatized by violence in the home tend to develop two characteristic sets of reactions. For boys the most common response is a state of constant vigilance, always on the lookout for "fight or flight." But for girls the more common reaction is dissociation, "disengaging from the external world *and attending to stimuli in the internal world*. . . . Children report 'going to a different place' . . . a sense of 'watching a movie that I was in,' or 'just floating.'" [Italics added]

Such "turning off," separating mentally from the immediate world around, doesn't have to be a sign of mental illness. Many of us go into a similar meditative state while driving a familiar road or performing other routine tasks. Early development of such meditative practices seems to lead to heightened psychic awareness. No wonder, then, that many more women than men become mediums or develop other outstanding psychic gifts. And that in many non-Western cultures, the child who easily drifts into trance is recruited for training as a medium or a shaman.*

When I discussed these theories with grown children of alcoholics after we'd completed our interviews, they came up with other ideas. Several women said that their substance-addicted fathers had a sensitive streak. Perhaps they drank to anesthetize themselves, to mute messages they didn't want to hear. Then a man who had worked for years as a medical technician in emergency rooms came up with a more detailed scientific hypothesis that drew on his knowledge of post-traumatic stress disorder (PTSD). According to Wayne,

> Hypervigilance states keep our fight or flight hormones going. These are called glucocorticoids. Hypervigilance states don't have to be about combat. They can be triggered by alcoholic parents or violent parents or by rape or incest, and actually the stress of working in emergency rooms—because you know that if you make an error, someone will die—now that's stress. And it's not just the combat, it's the waiting for combat, it's the waiting for a cardiac arrest to come in

---

*Just this process is described firsthand by the Dutch-born psychologist, Robert Wolff, in his artfully simple yet eloquent book, *What It Is to Be Human*. During the mid-twentieth century, Wolff visited often with the Sng'oi, aboriginal hunter-gatherers who lived in "high jungle" in the mountains of Malaysia. There he came to know and respect one of their shamans. After Wolff fell easily into trance at a Sng'oi ceremony, he was invited to study to be a shaman himself.

any minute now and you'll have to function or the person will die. And the waiting for it produces these glucocorticoids at levels continuously that they have found damaged the hippocampus in the brain.

Now the hippocampus is basically the key to memory. It sorts long-term memory, short-term memory, important memory. And in dead PTSD victims, they've found dead neurons in the hippocampus; and in live subjects, they found a shrinking of the hippocampus in relation to the post-traumatic stress disorder. It's actually poisoned by the glucocorticoids at high levels for long periods of time.

If long-term stress could trigger destructive physiological changes in adult brains, Wayne reasoned, perhaps in children's brains it could bring on more positive kinds of changes, modifications that empowered the child to take in information through psychic routes. Such a seemingly paradoxical outcome would not be all that unusual. After all, dexadrine, a stimulant for adults, can be used as a tranquilizer for children. Ritalin, widely prescribed to calm down hyperactive kids, is chemically similar to amphetamines.

It's been proven that childhood trauma can have strong long-term effects on chemical reactions in the brain. In a recent study done at the Mount Sinai School of Medicine in New York, women who had a history of childhood abuse were put in mildly stressful situations. They were asked to give a speech and to solve arithmetic problems in front of an audience. In response, according to *The New York Times,* they "showed levels of ACTH, a hormone secreted by the pituitary gland in response to stress, *six times as high* as those in women without such histories." [Emphasis added.] Mount Sinai's Traumatic Stress Studies Program has "documented abnormal stress responses in combat veterans, rape victims, survivors of the Holocaust and other who have endured traumatic experiences." Dr. Rachel Yehuda, director of the program, asserted that "the new study's findings support observations that our group has made over a 10-year period about the exquisite responsiveness of stress hormones in survivors who have sustained trauma in both childhood and adulthood."

The significant role of the pituitary gland in stress responses raises a tantalizing question. Oddly enough, this pea-sized gland located at the base of the brain is larger in women than in men. Its weight in men is only about half a gram but it can be twice as large in a woman who has had more than one child. (A slight increase in its size occurs during pregnancy, when it secretes prolactin, a hormone that among other things, stimulates breast development and formation of milk.) Now, women are more likely than men to show psychic powers. And widows are more likely than any other group to report contact with the dead experiences. They are also likely to have especially large pituitary glands since most of them have probably borne one or more children. Is it possible that this gland has some yet unidentified function in heightening sensitivity to psi?

Clearly, many influences interact to determine such sensitivity. Some of these are environmental, others genetic. Still others, for all we know, may be karmic or may carry over in some other way from a previous life. In my own research I've found a significant minority of psychics who reported that, during their childhoods, they experienced neither approval of psi nor any unusual trauma. This last is important and comforting. You *don't* have to be traumatized as a kid and you *don't* have to grow up in a pro-psi environment to develop psychic powers. What's more, even if you've never received psychic messages before, if you open your heart and mind, they'll probably come to you. When you least expect it some loving spirit will surprise you.

I speak from experience. In 1983 when my husband Paul died, I was well over forty. Over forty and determinedly rational, a skeptic about everything paranormal. Nonetheless, the vividness of my first communication from Paul and the fact that, mercifully, it came to my teenage son and me jointly, empowered me to begin to change my mind. The process snowballed. Because I was more open-minded, I was able to take in more messages—and that, in turn, made me more open-minded still.

One of my most thrilling psi experiences came over a decade after Paul's passing. For years I'd received messages from him—repeatedly though not often, sometimes with gaps of years between. But no other spirit presence ever brightened my door.

More and more I thought about my mother who'd made her transition in the fall of '64. At the time our relationship had been strained for quite a while. I'd chosen to live on the far side of the continent from her. Even after her passing, I often spoke of her critically. But as the years wore on, I started to see things in a different light. The pressures she'd put on me had made sense in their way. And she herself had had to survive pressures far more severe than any I'd ever endured. I longed to contact her spirit. I wondered: Should I search out a medium? But the skeptic in me still doubted mediums and I'd been spoiled by Paul who'd come to me directly. Then on April 28th of 1996, the first of two convincing manifestations occurred. This would have been my mother's one hundredth birthday; she was born exactly a century before.

On just that day I took a little walk around a side of my house where I rarely venture and discovered that on my neighbor's property, directly alongside my own, lilacs were growing—and lilacs were my mother's favorite flower. By then I'd lived in that house for over four years. How could I never have noticed this before? My mother's favorite flowers were blooming, sending their sweetness to me, tucked between other shrubs that had masked them before for me.

I keep a log of events I've experienced that seem paranormal. But before I make an entry in that log, I usually write a note to myself somewhere else so I can think about it for a while. Think about it, evaluate it, decide if it's really convincing. So I wrote a little note to myself on a yellow Post-it: "On mom's 100th birthday, discovered lilacs around back." I thought about it and thought about it—then decided not to transfer that note to my log. Because maybe, I thought, it was just a coincidence. I'm no botanist and not much of a gardener. Unless I passed by when the flowers were in bloom, I never would have spotted them. I tossed that Post-it in a waste basket somewhere.

But this was just the first of *two* manifestations. Exactly a year after I spotted those lilacs, I looked for them again. They weren't blooming. But on my desk, in plain sight, was that yellow Post-it. *That yellow Post-it that I'd thrown away.* And this manifestation was just like my mother. My mother was always afraid that the rest of us in the family would throw out something valuable, so she used to go through our waste baskets, just in case. At last I was convinced; I made an entry in my log.

My mother, God bless her, hadn't just come to answer my call. She'd taught me that, thirty-two years after her passing, some characteristic part of her lived on somewhere. In the next chapter we'll look at other valuable insights psychics have garnered from after-death contacts and other psi events.

17

Spiritual Experience and Religious Belief

DEALING WITH DEATH CAN BE SHATTERING. Dealing with survival of the spirit *after* death is a learning experience that lifts you up. It lifts you up while it challenges much you've been taught. It challenges you to rethink—and, perhaps, to reshape your life.

What skills I may have as a writer can't begin to convey the burning sincerity of the people I've interviewed, the glow of faces radiant with wonderment and exaltation. Sometimes the tales they told turned uproarious, sometimes weepy, often a bit of both. About a third of my informants, men as well as women, cried in the course of telling their stories.

Many said they'd been skeptics about survival before their after-death contacts but that personal experience had made them believers.

I raised both of my kids to question. Not to *not* believe, but to question anything because I'm the skeptic of all skeptics. I'm the person who says, "Really, that's true? Then prove it." Sometimes people kind of get off in woowoo land—you know, rampant paranormal things. I never believed them for a minute. Nobody was more surprised than I when that kind of thing occurred with me.

I think it's important for people to know about spirit. I couldn't believe in spirit unless I had experienced it. To me faith is shakier than experience. If someone says, "I believe this," maybe you can take that away. But if I experience it, no one can take that away from me. So I tell people about the experiences I've had because I think they're so heartening and it's important for people to know.

I'm old enough to remember when you had to believe what was in the Bible, you had to believe what the preacher said and the priest said. Other than that, we didn't know *what* happened after death. But when my grandmother came back to me in the most vivid dream I ever hope to have, it was proof to me that there was life after death and I wanted everybody to know. *[This dream was particularly convincing since the next morning the dreamer learned that her grandmother had died the previous night.]* I absolutely believe she didn't want us to worry. Ever since then I *know* there's life after death.

A number of my informants—whatever the faith, or lack of faith, they'd been raised in—were independent-minded, good-hearted folk who over time had journeyed to understandings which didn't fit conventional religious strictures. Several, for instance, mentioned that they had come to believe in reincarnation. Here's how one psychic, visiting in the States from New Zealand, described her beliefs.

I am one of the most profoundly religious people I know but one of the greatest problems I have is *organized* religion. I believe that the outrages that some religions have perpetrated on the world in the name of Jesus and God are the *true* sacrilege. But with every bone in my body, I believe there was a Jesus, I believe that he came to do the right thing. Just like Mohammed and Martin Luther King, Jr. and Mahatma Gandhi. They were all out there. They did their stuff. And spiritually I'm a great believer in Buddhism and I believe in reincarnation which, of course, *[laughing]* is at odds with organized religion too. There's a great thing that they say: the world's *real* religious leaders don't argue.

One of the amazing things that's going to happen in England when Prince Charles comes into power is that he's going to change it from "Defender of the Faith" to "Defender of the Faiths." Church and state will be separated. He's said that publicly.

Again and again, people that I interviewed rejected organized religion in similar terms.

I was raised Lutheran but I rebelled against it. I mean, I don't think of myself as a specifically religious person but more of a spiritual person.

I was raised Catholic. When I was 17 we had a parting of the ways. Right now I'm sort of on a spiritual quest. I don't consider myself to be a religious person, I don't believe in a particular religious philosophy, but I do consider myself to be a spiritual person.

Over the years I've become sort of a collage of Buddhist, Hindu, Spiritualist. *[Laughs]* I have tremendous respect for what specific religious leaders and specific people who follow certain religions do. I have very little respect for the parochialism or the rule-making that many of those religions have. I now view my church as being the world and I view action in a constructive way as the best kind of prayer.

I'm spiritual but not religious. My dad was a Christian mystic but he wasn't much of a churchgoer. I've always figured he had the right idea. His ideal and example was Jesus but he thought nobody was living that very well. If people really loved one another as they loved themselves then the whole world would be different. He tried his best to actually *live* that. Outcasts and rejects were welcome at our house. Everyone knew they could come to our place for help.

Sensing God in nature was a recurring theme among psychics. Other frequent comments recalled one of my favorite bumper stickers: God is too big to fit in any one religion.

When I was five, I asked my dad, "How big is God?" He says, "Well, look up at the stars. You'll learn about atoms when you get older but I'd say the stars are like the atoms in the body of God. And the whole universe would be how big God is."
. . . I believe there is this essential goodness in everyone. If they just lived that way, they wouldn't need all the complicated doctrines that tend to be more divisive than unitive. If you call God a different

name in different religions, then it seems like a different god when actually it's just a cultural language barrier. So it's the Nameless One as far as I'm concerned.

I am a third generation Unitarian. The church that I was very active in as a teenager was sort of: This is it, this is what we get. Ashes to ashes, dust to dust. There's nothing before and nothing after. But the experiences I've had are validation that probably the universe does work, everything's gonna fit.... It's not just about human beings. All the little life forms here and there and everywhere are all interconnected. And I believe that there is assistance from the other side. I think I have probably had a lot of assistance all my life. And only with a broader spiritual perspective am I aware of it and extremely grateful for it. So it's like a big happy family, not just people on this planet in human form.

My parents always taught us that spirit was within us and that we could go out in nature and be closer to God than in any church. Myself, I just started going from church to church, studied every church and I respect all of them. Love is the most important thing and I think it's at the heart of every religion. I pray to all the gods and goddesses.

It's no coincidence that the three great monotheistic religions of the world were formed in deserts, by desert people. And high altitude is very much like desert, because you don't have many trees. There are great visual effects there, lots and lots of sky. The very deep blue skies and the very twisted trees that have taken such strength to survive in such areas have been like religious icons to me. Joshua trees. Some very, very old trees in the Sierras. Something that's been alive for 2,000 years and is still alive and reproducing has a lot of wisdom. It deserves a lot of respect. I've sat and meditated with trees like that. Most of my major decisions during the past twenty years of my life I've made in the Sierras or the high desert or some other what I would call very spiritual place.

By contrast, a number of other psychics reported that contact experiences with departed spirits had strengthened their allegiance to their chosen religion.

[*From a deacon in the Episcopal Church*] I feel as if my life has been guided and sometimes I've gone kicking and screaming. But that God is God is no problem to me. And God becomes more and more. You can call God any name you need and God will lead and guide and direct and encourage. But when you say there is no god, God's, shall we say, hands are tied. You have to be open to receive. It's as if faith is the conduit, it goes both ways.

I was raised Catholic and I thought I had a certain amount of strong faith—until the experience after I lost my dad [*sensing his presence and seeing a light turn itself on*] made it so much more of a known to me. Before I had a faith that there was a God and the rest of it, but now I just know. There's no question anymore in my mind, if there ever was.

Another experience, coming from *beyond* the dead, was when Dad was ill. A missionary came to our church that was praying specifically for the ill. So I went to a service and the Eucharist was exposed and I was praying pretty intensely that he was going to recover. And I felt a sensation start at the top of my head and go all the way through me. A tingle. And I've never, ever experienced anything like that or ever thought that I would. I was able to talk to my dad about it. He said, "Wow, that was through me that that happened to you, which is so wonderful." Because he'd always had that knowledge, that deep, deep faith.

[*From a Methodist*] Every night, after we'd get through eating supper, we'd take out the Bible and read it. I always felt God was there, God was near us. He's got a very soft voice and you know it when you hear it, and he's always been that close to me. Of course everything I told my husband that I'd learned from the Lord, he never believed until afterwards. He'd ask me, "How'd you know?" God said he didn't want anyone to be ignorant. I've always felt you have to have that childlike faith.

Contact experiences give us brief glimpses of the other side. Unexpectedly, as if in a darkened theater, curtains part. Someone we've loved is lit by the flare of a spotlight that illumines a fragment of their afterlife world. Then darkness again. But images remain, scant but stunningly vivid, to hold in our hearts and maybe puzzle over. To analyze—but not to analyze *away*. Contact experiences teach us many things:

- Some essential part of us can be immortal or at least can survive for decades after death.

- Spirits move on to another place. Most seem to be happy there.

- Contact experiences with the dead are usually expressions of love or at least of concern for the welfare of the living.

- Like near-death experiences, ADCs tend to engender heightened unselfishness and an intensification of spiritual values.

The messages most frequently received from the other side are, "Don't worry about me. I'm okay," (or "I'm happy now,") and "Stop grieving for me. Get on with your life." Sometimes these are accompanied by a promise like, "I'll always love you and watch over you." Messages like these encourage the living to make the most of their earthly adventure. At the same time they reassure us that for the great majority of those who die, death is neither a final end nor the beginning of some frightening ordeal.

What they do *not* tell us is that all who die face the same fate. (The fact that only a fraction of those who come back from clinical death report a classic "near-death experience" suggests the same thing.) Three patterns in the ADCs I've heard of suggest that, in fact, spirits can travel quite different routes after death.

- Often a sensitive who has received numerous messages from one parent, will never receive any at all from the other. Or someone who has sensed contact with several lost loved ones will wonder aloud why they have never heard from some particular beloved who has passed on. Does lack of communication simply indicate a lack of interest on the other side? Or is that spirit being held beyond reach, out of touch for a time with its former fellows?

- Several people reported contacts with spirits who wanted to apologize for their past misbehavior. In Chapter 7 we met four women who told stories of an erring parent who came back to reach out to a daughter they'd hurt or shortchanged in life. Was this the result of something they learned after death? Or a condition they had to satisfy to move on to something better?

- What happens after death to the really evil? To murderers, for example? Three of my interviewees reported contact experiences with murder victims but nobody reported contact with a murderer. The literature of the paranormal is loaded with accounts of ADCs with people who committed suicide—I myself have collected many—but, although I've sought advice from numerous researchers on spirit survival, I have yet to locate a single spontaneous after-death communication from the spirit of someone who murdered someone else. A landmark study, based on descriptions of ADCs from 2,000 men, women and children, noted that "to our knowledge, no one who was interviewed was contacted by anybody who had committed malicious crimes or atrocities."

In a recent book Michael Newton describes what may happen after death to the souls of people with exceptionally cruel life styles. Dr. Newton is a licensed hypnotherapist who uses age-regression techniques to study the experiences of souls *between* incarnations. Improbable as this research may sound, I'm inclined to view it with interest since many of Newton's findings jibe with those of responsible researchers who study related issues in less unorthodox ways. Interviewing a subject whom he had regressed under hypnosis to a post-death state—a subject said to be in training to deal with "atrocity souls"—Newton was told that "if we think they are salvageable, they are offered a choice to come back to Earth in roles where they will receive the same type of pain they caused, only multiplied. . . . It usually will take more than one life to endure an equal measure of the same kind of pain they caused to many people."

One of the most startling stories I've recorded strongly suggests the existence of some place of enforced, therapeutic, solitary meditation for troubled spirits who have committed lesser misdeeds. This contact experience came about in a complicated fashion. First Lisa, a skilled health professional who is very sensitive to psi, found a ouija board.

My mother's brother died fairly young. He had a daughter who'd been living in Japan but was in the States visiting. My cousin's last full day here before she left, she wanted to go shopping. I really don't like to shop but I did want to spend quality time with her and my sister. She was staying with my sister in Maryland and I was living in DC. So I made a deal with her that I'd bring my bike along with me on my car so I could go to the park while she and my sister cooked dinner. It was important for me to be in nature 'cause I lived and worked in the city during the week.

So we spent the day shopping and as soon as we got back to my sister's house, they went in to start preparing dinner and I got the bike off my car. To get to the park by my sister's house was a left turn and then another left turn. So I got on the bike with a full intention of going to the corner and making a left but all of a sudden from my solar plexus area there was a tug and I was compelled to make a right turn. [*A series of other unexpected impulses led her not to the park that had been her destination but to a tiny bridge over a creek. There Lisa stopped, still straddling her bike.*]

I'm looking down and I'm remembering this creek from my childhood. I couldn't go forward because there was a box in front of the tire. It was broad daylight but I hadn't noticed it before. So I look at it and it's a ouija board box. Okay, I figure, it's just the lid, must've blown here from someone's garbage. So I bent down, lifted it up with my finger and it was a whole ouija board and the thing looked brand new. Well, I've had enough strange experiences in my past to know, "Okay," so I picked it up and put it on the back of my bike and pedaled home to my sister's house. [*When her sister saw the ouija board, she chose to keep working in the kitchen. But Lisa's cousin was intrigued.*]

She instantly sat down with me. I told her how it worked, and we started to ask it questions. Now the strange thing about it was, every single question we asked it, instantly got a dynamic, perfectly clear response. Usually you wait for it to move over to this letter and you wait, you know, for the next letter. This was just like boom boom boom boom boom, to all the letters. We weren't writing things down—we were just playing at this point. But my cousin kept throwing her arms up. She'd get goosebumps and say, "You're doing that, you're doing that." And I said, "Kathy, I'm not doing that. Even if I was pushing it in your direction which I could do, how could I pull it in *my* direction?" It was going so fast we could hardly keep our fingers on it, that's how fast it was moving.

We were asking it stupid questions like where am I going to live? And who am I gonna marry? And what am I gonna do for a living? But when I asked it what I was gonna do for a living it cracked me up because it spelled out "dysfunction" and at this point I was on my way to go back to school to study alcohol and drug counseling. So it occurred to me for some reason to say, "Maybe this is *somebody*." So I said, "Who are you?" and it spelled out right away, "Kathy's dad."

Well, my cousin just freaked out. She's always been very Polly-anna, she acts like there's no dark side. She said something like, "Are you happy? Are you in a good place?" And he said, "No." I mean, there were just so many answers in what happened that never would've been *our* answers.

So he said, "No," and she said, "Why not?" And he wrote out, "It's lonely here." And then I said to him, "Where are you?" And this was really out of left field 'cause neither one of us would've said this. He said, "The underworld." And you know, when I look back at it, in retrospect, if there is such a thing as an underworld, which neither of us really believed in, my uncle would've qualified [laughs] to go there.

His mother died when he was eight. After that he was pretty much a street urchin, smoking cigarettes and drinking instead of going to school. And then his whole life. He got married. He had four kids. But he philandered with other women. He was never a good provider. He threw his money away on alcohol. On cigarettes and gambling and other women. He had a great sense of humor and I think he had a good heart but he was extremely dysfunctional. It was just all of that drama ... he left his wife for a younger woman. Everybody liked him, he was very social. He just wasn't a good adult. So anyway.

He said, "the underworld" and that freaked my cousin out. So then she said, "Why are you here? Are you going to come back to Japan with me?" And he said, "No." And she said, "What did you come to say?" And he spells out. . . . I didn't know what this meant until she burst into tears, but the ouija board spelled out, "Love to love ya, Kel." And their last name is Kelly. And that had been something private between them, what he used to say to her, "Love to love ya, Kel." And she instantly burst into tears and went hysterical.

The next day, the ouija board looked ratty because somebody had used it. Where before, it hadn't looked used at all. And the people in the household were trying to play with it but it never really worked for them the way it had worked for us. Because it really wasn't *us*, you know, it was definitely him talking. He was using it as a vehicle to speak.

The thing that I found interesting in retrospect was even if there is an underworld, it's not what we think it is. Cause the fact is, he could still come back, he still had some kind of power to make this whole thing happen just so he could come say, "I love you" to his daughter.

Here then is yet another parent seeking reconciliation with a daughter. Were the other four visiting from some underworld too? The visiting spirit's remark about feeling lonely recalls Summer's account back in Chapter 2 about dreams she had for years of her mother that suggested to her that her mother's spirit was "kind of lost. I'm not sure she knew she was dead in the beginning. Like she would come back and sneak around and look around the corner at us. And she was alone and I'd try to bring her into the living room and she would start crying and say no. We were worried about her being in pain and we couldn't help her, her being lonely." Fortunately, when Summer's grandmother died ten years after the death of her daughter (Summer's mother), the two of them appeared together to Summer to reassure her that they were both doing fine in the afterlife. Had her mother finally graduated and moved on to more joyous fields?

These stories also recall a "realm of bewildered spirits" described by Raymond Moody. Soon after publication of his bestselling book, *Life after Life*, which introduced millions to the quintessential near-death experience, Moody—who by now had interviewed still more NDE survivors—added to his original list of typical features of the near-death experience, a few less common elements. Generally these elements had been reported to him by people whose forays into clinical death had lasted particularly long.

In *Reflections on Life after Life,* Dr. Moody reported that several survivors had glimpsed "dulled spirits" in a gray, washed out area. Their heads were bent downwards; they seemed sad and depressed. A woman who had been believed dead for 15 minutes said they seemed to be "searching, but for what they were searching I don't know. . . . They seemed to be caught in between somewhere. . . . They may have some contact with the physical world. Something is tying them down, because they all seemed to be bent over and looking downward, maybe into the physical world . . . maybe watching something they hadn't done or should do."

According to Moody, several informants "noticed certain of these beings trying unsuccessfully to communicate with people who were still physically alive. One man . . . saw an ordinary man walking, unaware, while one of these dulled spirits hovered above him. He said he had the feeling that this spirit had been, while alive, the man's mother, and, still unable to give up her earthly role, was trying to tell her son what to do. . . ." A second woman informant described spirits trying unsuccessfully to contact the living.

> They were trying to communicate, yet there was no way they could break through. . . .
>
> One seemed to be a woman who was trying so hard to reach through to children and to an older woman in the house. . . . She was trying to get them to do the right things, to change so as not to be left like she was. . . . "Do things for others so that you won't be left like this. . . ."

These accounts of the realm of bewildered spirits recall pictures which many faiths have drawn of the afterlife. In different ways they bear some resemblance to the She'ol of the ancient Hebrews, to ancient Greek notions of exile beyond the river Styx, and to the Zoroastrian limbo that awaited those judged to have been neither particularly good nor bad in life. They also suggest the redemption through suffering of purgatory. It seems more than likely that time and again over thousands of years, mystics, psychics and survivors of close calls with death have envisioned just such a realm.

I'm reminded of a stylish woman, successful in a competitive career, who made some wise comments about issues like these. Jan is intensely psychic. After I had finished my interview with her, she started out my front door, then turned abruptly and asked me, "Are you an Aquarius or a Gemini?" I gasped—then acknowledged that I was an Aquarius. Smiling, she said, "I *know* things like that." Here's what she said about speculating about the immediate fates of those who "shuffle off this mortal coil."

> There was a time when I tried to read things into how long was it between when a person died and when I heard from them. I wondered, was that significant in some way? Did it mean that they were in some other place first? Why didn't I hear sooner? And I finally just said, That part's not important.
>
> I think we keep getting presented with something over and over again until we get the message. I believe that there are spirits around us at all times. Some people call them angels, I don't know. I don't think that when I die that my spirit is going to go to a *place* but I would find it really hard to believe that when we die we just die. We die *physically* but I think there's a *spiritual* part of us that lives on.

Clearly over the years, many a message has come to psychics to help them envision what may await us on the other side. Happily, much of what they tell us is heartening and joyous. Their sense of the world we live in—the *totality* of the world and our existence— is many-sided and beautiful.

> I think actual physical death is just, if not an illusion, it's just one of those things that happen. I think there's a definite continuity in my spirit, your spirit, everybody's spirit. They've just changed form.

> I have a better relationship with my father than I ever did when he was alive. Now that he's not on this plane and constricted by his own physical humanness, I feel him in my own actions. His presence is being distilled into me, as a shot of booster energy to me.

> Life does not stop when you die. The bodies we have are just like husks or vehicles. They're not the soul, they have nothing to do with the soul. And the soul does not die.

What does this vision of the human condition mean for us here? I think that answer was given best by a pretty strawberry blonde in her thirties. Kerry was born into a family of clairvoyants: one grandmother told fortunes with cards, the other read tea leaves. She is also the daughter of an alcoholic mother and a father with a violent, hair-trigger temper. A natural medium, she never charges for her services. Often she receives messages from departed spirits for those they left behind.

> It's really important that people understand that there's more to life than money. The world is in a very bad place. I'm not happy with it. I'm blessed that I have this ability and I hope that it can help people. Part of it is knowing that you never ever die wishing you had more money. You die wishing that you'd loved more or that you'd been kinder. Those are the things that they often will pass on to me to tell people. And hindsight is 20-20 and they know. They get to sit up there and know the mistakes they've made. It's not easy when you go up there with a lot of regrets.

No doubt, knee-jerk disbelievers will discount judgments like these as the fantasies of deluded folk. Afraid that they will be confused by facts, they close their minds to evidence like that presented here. But if this book convinces at least a few thoughtful skeptics that messages can reach us from the other side, if it heartens some of the multitude who have received such messages to share their stories with their neighbors, then these pages will have been well worth writing.

Throughout the millennia, humans around the globe have turned to sensitives to penetrate the veil of death and teach them high wisdom. Today's scientists have developed awesome skills for weighing and analyzing material things but so far they've failed to detect the fine, essential stuff of spirit. Perhaps someday they will find it—but first they will have to shed their prejudices and preconceived notions. For the open-minded it should be clear that spirit exists.

Notes

CHAPTER 1

Page 4—Sir Oliver Lodge: Lodge, O. (1916) *Raymond; or Life and death, with examples of the survival of memory and affection after death*. New York: George H. Doran.

Page 8—European Human Values Study: Harding, S., Phillips, D., with Fogarty, M. (1986) *Contrasting values in Western Europe: unity, diversity, and change*. London: Macmillan. Cited in: Haraldson, E. "Survey of claimed encounters with the dead." (1988) *Omega* 19 (2) 103-113.

    Mourning in Japan: Yamamoto, J., Okonogi, K., Iwasaki, T., and Yoshimura, S. (1969) "Mourning in Japan." *American Journal of Psychiatry*. 125, 1660-65.

Page 9—Welsh study: Rees, W. D. (1971) "The Hallucinations of widowhood." *British Medical Journal*. 4, 37-41.

    Los Angeles survey: Kalish, R. A., and Reynolds, D. K. (1973) "Phenomenological reality and post-death contact." *Journal for the Scientific Study of Religion*. 12 (2) 209-21.

Page 10—Harvard Bereavement Study: Parkes, C.M., and Weiss, R. S. (1983) *Recovery from bereavement*. New York: Basic Books.

    Teenagers who lost a sibling: Balk, D. (1983) "Adolescents' grief reactions and self-concept perceptions following sibling death: a study of 33 teenagers." *Journal of Youth and Adolescence*. 12 (2) 137-61.

North Carolina widows and widowers: Olson, P. R., Suddeth, J. A., Peterson, P. J., and Egelhoff, C. (1985) "Hallucinations of widowhood." *Journal of the American Geriatric Association.* 33, 543-47.

Page 11—Polling data, National Opinion Research Center: Greeley, A. M. (1989) *Religious change in America.* Cambridge, MA: Harvard University Press.

Young adults who lost parents: Meshot, C. M. and Leitner, L. M. (1993) "Adolescent mourning and parental death." *Omega* 26, 4, 287-299.

Swedish study: Grimby, A. (1993) "Bereavement among elderly people: grief reactions, post-bereavement hallucinations and quality of life." *Acta psychiatrica Scandinavica* 87 (1) 72-80.

Page 12 —Norwegian study: Lindstrom, T. C. (1995) "Experiencing the presence of the dead: discrepancies in 'the sensing experience' and their psychological concomitants." *Omega* 31, 1, 11-21.

Study of Massachusetts widows: Conant, R. D. (1992) *Widow's experiences of intrusive memory and "sense of presence" of the deceased after sudden and untimely death of a spouse during mid-life.* Doctoral dissertation, Massachusetts School of Professional Psychology, West Roxbury, MA.

Books by Louis E. LaGrand: (1998) *After-death communication; final farewells.* St. Paul, MN: Llewellyn Publications; (1999) *Messages and miracles; extraordinary experiences of the bereaved.* St. Paul, MN: Llewellyn Publications.

Talking to Heaven: van Praagh, J. (1997) *Talking to heaven: a medium's message of life after death.* New York: Dutton.

Hello from Heaven!: Guggenheim, B., and Guggenheim, J. (1995) *Hello from heaven!* New York: Bantam.

Page 13—Greeley on need for in-depth interviews: Greeley, A. M. (1975) *The sociology of the paranormal: a reconnaissance.* Beverly Hills/London: Sage Publications.

In-depth interviews by S. H. Wright: For a more scholarly report on the author's interview methods and findings, see: Wright, S. H. (1999) "Paranormal contact with the dying: 14 contemporary death coincidences." *Journal of the Society for Psychical Research.* 63 (857) 258-267.

CHAPTER 2

Page 16—Song, "Grandfather's clock": "Grandfather's clock." (1876) Words and music by H. C. Work. Numerous editions.

Page 18—Duke data on spontaneous events: Rhine, L. E. (1963) "Spontaneous physical effects and the psi process." *Journal of Parapsychology.* 27:84-122.

Page 19—Second sight: Cohn, S. A. (1999) "A questionnaire study of second sight experiences." *Journal of the Society for Psychical Research.* 63, 129-157. This valuable recent study lists other useful works on this subject by Cohn.
    Further data on death coincidences: Wright, S. H. (1999).

Page 22—Traditional Jewish tale: Buber, M. (1977) *Tales of the Hasidim.* Volume 2. New York: Schocken Books. Quoted in: Raphael, S. P. (1994) *Jewish Views of the Afterlife.* Northvale, NJ and London: Jason Aronson, Inc.

Page 28—Census of Hallucinations: Sidgwick, H., Johnson, A., Myers, A.T. (deceased at time of report's preparation), Podmore, F., and Sidgwick, E. ("Prof. Sidgwick's Committee") (1894) Report on the Census of Hallucinations. *Proceedings of the Society for Psychical Research.* 10, 25-422.

CHAPTER 4

Page 47—Cross-cultural study on grief and mourning: Rosenblatt, P.C., Walsh, R. P., and Jackson, D. A. (1976) *Grief and mourning in cross-cultural perspective.* HRAF Press [USA: Human Relations Area Files, Inc.]

Page 48—Trobriand Islanders: Malinowski, B. (1929) *The sexual life of savages in North-Western Melanesia.* New York: Halcyon House.

Page 50—Funeral practices of Gauls, Celts, etc.: Ries, J. (1987) "Immortality" in Eliade, M., ed. *Encyclopedia of Religion.* New York: Macmillan.

Slavic folk beliefs: Mansikka, V. J. (1955) "Demons and spirits (Slavic)," in *Encyclopaedia of Religion and Ethics*, v. 4. Hastings, J., ed. New York: Charles Scribner's Sons.

Shamanism in Siberia: Keleman, M., reporting. (August 18, 1999) Morning Edition, National Public Radio. Transcript produced by Burrelle's Information Services, Livingston, New Jersey.

Page 51—Mari practices: Ries, J. (1987)

Kikuyu practices: Kenyatta, J. (1978) *Facing Mt. Kenya; the tribal life of the Gikuyu.* New York: AMS Press.

African practices: Lawson, E. T. (1985) *Religions of Africa; traditions in transformation.* New York: Harper & Row.

Page 52—Educated Africans: Boshier, A. (1976) "The religions of Africa" in Toynbee, A., Koestler, A., and others. *Life after death.* New York: McGraw-Hill; Olupona, J.K., ed. (1991) *African traditional religion in contemporary society.* New York: Paragon House.

Yoruban practices in the Western hemisphere: Guiley, R. E. (1991) *Harper's encyclopedia of mystical & paranormal experience.* San Francisco: HarperSanFrancisco.

Ancient Egyptian and Mesopotamian beliefs: Ries, J. (1987)

Page 53—Ancient Greek festival: Crehan, J. (1976) "Near Eastern societies," in Toynbee, A., Koestler, A. and others. *Life after death.* New York: McGraw-Hill.

Grave marker on Rhodes: Copied by the author in 1997 from an exhibit at the archeological museum on the island of Rhodes.

Roman festival of Parentalia: Crehan, J. (1976)

Page 54—Ancient Israelite burial practices: Raphael, S. P. (1996) *Jewish views of the afterlife.* Northvale: New Jersey and London: Jason Aronson, Inc.

Ancient Islamic beliefs: Seale, M. S. (1976) "Islamic society," in Toynbee, A., Koestler, A. and others. *Life after death.* New York: McGraw-Hill.

Page 55—Zoroastrians: Boyce, M. (1987) *Zoroastrians; their religious beliefs and practices.* London: Routledge & Kegan Paul.

Page 57—Pivotal Jewish thinkers: Raphael, S. P. (1996)

Page 59—1994 Gallup poll: Gallup, G., Jr. (1995) *The Gallup poll; public opinion 1994.* Wilmington, Delaware: Scholarly Resources, Inc.

1998 Gallup poll: Gallup, G., Jr. (1999) *The Gallup Poll; public opinion 1998.* Wilmington, Delaware: Scholarly Resources, Inc.

CHAPTER 5

Page 63—Joe McMoneagle: McMoneagle, J. (1997) *Mind trek; exploring consciousness, time, and space through remote viewing.* Charlottesville, VA: Hampton Roads Publishing.

Page 64—Orloff on mainstream physicians: Orloff, J. (1996) *Second sight.* New York: Warner Books.

Characteristics of shamans: Walsh, R. (1990) *The spirit of shamanism.* New York: G.P. Putnam's Sons.

Mental health of mystics: Greeley, A. (1975) *The Sociology of the paranormal: a reconnaissance.* Beverly Hills: Sage Publications.

Page 65—Hand washing by physicians: "Doctors are reminded, wash up!" *New York Times.* 9 November 1999: Page D1 in national edition, F1 in local edition.

Views of medical-scientific establishment on psi: Gallup, G., Jr., with Proctor, W. (1882) *Adventures in immortality.* New York: McGraw-Hill.

Page 66—Survey of 2700 physicians: Greeley, A. "Physician's religion as clinical asset." Unpublished report.

Research on healing power of prayer: Targ, R. and Katra, J. (1998) *Miracles of mind: exploring nonlocal consciousness and spiritual healing.* Novato, CA: New World Library; de Carvalho, M. M. (1996) "An eclectic approach to group healing in Sao Paulo, Brazil: a pilot study." *Journal of the Society for Psychical Research* 61, 845, 243-250.

Dossey on Spindrift and power of prayer: *Larry Dossey in conversation with Michael Toms.* (1994) New Dimensions Books. Lower Lake, California: Aslan Publishing.

Moody on scientific skeptics: Moody, R. (1999) *The last laugh; a new philosophy of near-death experiences, apparitions, and the paranormal.* Charlottesville, VA: Hampton Roads Publishing.

Page 67—DNA and tree of life: Stevens, W. K. (August 31, 1999) "Rearranging the branches on a new tree of life." *The New York Times*, D1.

Page 68—Boyce on the Zoroastrians: Boyce, M. (1987)

Page 69—Shamanic wisdom: Davis, W. (1998) *Shadows in the sun: travels to landscapes of spirit and desire.* Washington, DC: Island Press. Further interesting comments on the wisdom of indigenous shamans appear in Dr. Mark J. Plotkin's letter, "Mission in the rain forest." (*New York Times*, December 12, 1999, page 2 of the Science Times section.) Plotkin is president of the Amazon Conservation Team.

Page 70—Remen on one physician's inspired choice of a remedy: Remen, R. N. (1996) *Kitchen table wisdom: stories that heal.* New York: Riverhead Books.

Page 73—Study by Welsh physician: Rees, W. D. (1971) "The hallucinations of widowhood." *British Medical Journal*, 4, 37.

MacGregor on the Christian theological tradition: MacGregor, G. (1987) "Soul: Christian concept." In M. Eliade, editor in chief, *Encyclopedia of Religion.* New York : Macmillan.

Page 74—Haynes on the Reformation: Haynes, R. (1976) "Some Christian imagery." In A. Toynbee, A. Koestler, and others. *Life after death.* New York: McGraw-Hill.

Page 75—Jehovah's Witnesses: What hope for dead loved ones. (1987) New York: Watchtower Bible and Tract Society.

Days of the Dead: The days of the dead. (n.d.) Chicago: Mexican Fine Arts Museum.

Halloween: Primiano, L. N. (1987) "Halloween." In M. Eliade, editor in chief, *Encyclopedia of Religion.* New York: Macmillan.

Page 76—Religious beliefs of Americans: CNN/USA *Today*/Gallup Poll, interviewing dates 12/16-18/94. Gallup, G., Jr. (1995) *The Gallup Poll; public opinion 1994.* Wilmington, Delaware: Scholarly Resources, Inc.

CHAPTER 8

Page 109—Identical twins: Playfair, G. L. (1999) "Telepathy and identical twins." *Journal of the Society for Psychical Research*, 63, 854, 86-98.

CHAPTER 9

Page 115—1909 book by Sir Oliver Lodge: Lodge, O. (1909) *The survival of man; a study in unrecognized human faculty.* New York: Moffat, Yard.

Page 116—1916 book by Lodge: Lodge, O. (1916) *Raymond; or Life and death, with examples of the evidence for survival of memory and affection after death.* New York: George H. Doran.

CHAPTER 10

Page 126—William Barrett and the SPR: Beloff, J. (1993) *Parapsychology: a concise history.* New York: St. Martin's Press.

Lodge's scientific work, etc.: Ferguson, A. (1949) *Dictionary of national biography, 1931-1940.* London: Oxford University Press.

Flammarion's 3-volume study: Flammarion, C. (1921-23) *Death and its mystery.* Vol. 1: *Before death;* vol. 2: *At the moment of death;* vol. 3: *After death.* New York: The Century Co. Related books by Flammarion available in English include *The unknown* (New York: Harper, 1901) and *Haunted houses* (New York: Appleton, 1924.)

Page 127—T. H. Huxley on the scientific attitude: Quoted in: Huxley, L. A. (1968) *This timeless moment: a personal view of Aldous Huxley.* New York: Farrar, Straus & Giroux, p. 330.

Page 132—Roberta Conant's Study: Conant, R. D. (1992)

Page 133—Book by Bishop Pike: Pike, J. A., with Kennedy, D. (1968) *The other side: an account of my experiences with psychic phenomena.* Garden City, NY: Doubleday. This is a truly extraordinary document written by a man who made a fetish of his own rationality.

CHAPTER 12

Page 153—Drawings of butterflies in a concentration camp: Kübler-Ross, E. (1997) *The Wheel of Life: a memoir of living and dying.* New York: Scribner.

CHAPTER 14

Page 174—Psychokinetic stunts in Soviet Union: Gris, H. and Dick, W. (1978) *The new Soviet psychic discoveries.* Englewood Cliffs, NJ: Prentice-Hall.

Page 180—Types of poltergeist phenomena: Stevenson, I. (1972) "Are poltergeists living or are they dead?" *Journal of the American Society for Psychical Research.* 66, 3: 233-252.

CHAPTER 16

Page 195—CBS poll: CBS News Poll, April 20-22, 1998. Data supplied by the Roper Center, University of Connecticut.

An earlier poll: Greeley, A. M. (1975) *The Sociology of the Paranormal.* Beverly Hills/London: Sage Publications.

Table 1: Haraldsson, E. (1985) "Representative national surveys of psychic phenomena; Iceland, Great Britain, Sweden, U.S.A. and Gallup's multinational survey." *Journal of the Society for Psychical Research.* 53, 801, 145-158.

Page 197—Identical twins: Playfair, G. L. (1999) "Identical twins and telepathy." *Journal of the Society for Psychical Research.* 63, 854, 86-98.

Page 198—Kulagina and telekinesis: Gris, H., and Dick, W. (1978)

Emmons on upbringing of mediums: Emmons, C. F. (1998) Socialization to spirit mediumship. Address delivered to the Eastern Sociological Society, March 21, 1998.

Second sight in Scotland: Cohn, S. A. (1999A) "Second sight and family history: pedigree and segregation analyses." *Journal of Scientific Exploration.* 13, 3, 351-372.

Cohn, S. A. (1999B) "A historical review of second sight: the collectors, their accounts and ideas. *Scottish Studies.* 33, 146-185.

Cohn, S. A. (1999C) "A questionnaire study on second sight experiences." *Journal of the Society for Psychical Research*, 63, 855, 129-157.

Page 200—Alcoholism in America: National Council on Alcoholism and Drug Dependence. (1998) Alcoholism and alcohol-related problems: a sobering look. Fact sheet downloaded from www.ncadd.org.

Page 201—Schwarz and Perry on stress: Schwarz, E. D. and Perry, B. D. (1994) "The post-traumatic response in children and adolescents." *Psychiatric Clinics of North America*, 17, 2, 311-326.

Page 203—Steiger on mediums: Steiger, B. (1982) *The world beyond death.* Norfolk, VA: Downing Company.
    1973 sociological study on psychic experiences, etc.: The NORC-Luce Foundation Basic Belief Study, conducted by the National Opinion Research Center, the University of Chicago, in the winter and spring of 1973; Greeley, A. M. (1975) *The sociology of the paranormal: a reconnaissance.* Beverly Hills/London: Sage Publications.

Page 204—Lawrence on trauma and psychic experience: Lawrence, T., Edwards, C., Barraclough, N., Church, S. and Hetherington, F. (1995) "Modelling childhood causes of paranormal belief and experience: childhood trauma and childhood fantasy. *Personality & Individual Differences*, 19, 2, 207-215.
    Lawrence, T. Paranormal experience and the traumatized mind. Address to the Society for Psychical Research, London, May 13, 1999.

Page 205—Neurologists on the brain during a child's first years: "Fertile minds." *Time* (cover story) 149, 5: 49-56.
    Learning a foreign language: Birdsong, D., ed. (1999) *Second language acquisition and the critical period hypothesis.* Mahwah, NJ: Lawrence Erlbaum Associates.
    Acquiring absolute pitch: Ward, W. D . (1999) "Absolute pitch," in Deutsch, D., ed. *The Psychology of Music.* 2nd ed. San Diego: Academic Press.
    Reactions to violent trauma: Perry, B. D. and Pollard, R. (1998) "Homeostasis, stress, trauma, and adaptation: a neurodevelopmental view of childhood trauma." *Child and Adolescent Psychiatric Clinics of North America* 7, 33-51.

Page 206—Drifting easily into trance: Wolff, R. (1994) *What it is to be human.* Freeland, WA: Periwinkle Press.

Page 207—Post-traumatic stress disorder: Useful works on this complex subject include: Wilson, J. P., Harel, Z., and Kahana, B., eds. (1988) *Human adaptation to extreme stress: from the Holocaust to Vietnam.* NY: Plenum; Yehuda, R., ed. (1998) *Psychological trauma.* Washington, DC: American Psychiatric Press; Henry, J. P. (1993) "Psychological and physiological responses to stress: the right hemisphere and the hypothalamo-pituitary-adrenal axis, an inquiry into problems of human bonding." *Integrative Physiological and Behavioral Science,* 28, 4:369-387. Also of interest is: Davis, L. L., Clark, D. M., Kramer, G. L., Moeller, F. G., and Petty, F. (1999) "D-fenfluramine challenge in posttraumatic stress disorder," *Biological Psychiatry,* 45, 928-930. This brief article alerts the reader to abnormalities which male veterans suffering from PTSD experience in their secretion of prolactin. Diminished secretion of prolactin appears to be associated with heightened symptoms of PTSD and aggression. Prolactin is produced in the pituitary gland.

    Response to stress by survivors of childhood abuse: Goode, E. (2000) "Childhood abuse and adult stress; a study links trauma, depression and response to anxiety." *The New York Times,* August 1, 2000, A14.

Page 208—Anatomy of the pituitary gland: Gray, H. (1985) *Anatomy of the human body.* 30th American ed. C. D. Clemente, ed. Philadelphia: Lea & Febiger; Nolte, J. (1999) *The human brain: an introduction to its functional anatomy.* 4th ed. St. Louis, MO: Mosby.

CHAPTER 17

Page 217—A landmark study of ADCs: Guggenheim, B, and Guggenheim, J. (1995)

    Newton on "atrocity souls": Newton, M. (2000) *Destiny of souls.* St. Paul, MN: Llewellyn Publications.

Page 221—Moody on "dulled spirits": Moody, R. (1977) *Reflections on Life after life.* Harrisburg, PA: Stackpole Books.

Index

AIDS, 21, 66, 82-83

African traditional religions, 51-52

after-death communication [ADC], earlier research studies
- college students, 11
- comforting nature, 9
- not related to depression, 9
- not related to social isolation, 9
- parent, sensing a deceased, 11
- sibling, sensing a deceased, 10
- teenagers, 10-11
- widows and widowers, 1, 9-12, 194-195, 208

after-death communication, implications, 215-223

after-death communication, most common messages, 216

after-death communication, research around the world
- France, 195
- Iceland, 8, 195
- Italy, 8, 195
- Japan, 1, 9
- Norway, 1, 12
- Sweden, 1, 11
- United Kingdom, 1, 8, 195
- United States, 9-12, 76, 195
- West Germany, 8, 195

after-death communication, routes for
- animal behavior, anomalous, 15, 111, 149-158, 181

apparitions, 14, 19-21, 78, 80-83, 86, 153-155, 157-158, 162-163, 172-173, 175-177 (See also visions)

darkness as an omen of death, 21-22, 99

dreams, 4, 14, 24-26, 39-40, 48, 72-73, 78, 80-81, 84-86, 88, 97-100, 105-107, 139, 143, 157, 160-161, 164, 167-168, 181, 188-193

electrical devices aside from lights, 6, 12, 114, 117-118, 124-134

flowers and other plants, 143, 209

grief, feelings of, as a premonition, 23-24

hearing, 14, 23, 36, 43, 85-86, 100, 110-111, 130, 156-159, 169, 173, 181

kinesthetic experiences, 26-27, 81-82, 156-157, 169

lights, electrical, 3-7, 12, 14, 41-42, 86-87, 115-123

lights, not electrical, 21, 107-108, 138, 165, 191, 197-198

music, 143-144, 147, 149, 197

ouija boards, 133-134, 218-220

physical objects, odd behavior of, 6-8, 14, 16-19, 23, 64-65, 95-96, 108-109, 111-112, 133, 136-147, 161, 166, 170-171, 174-175,

after-death communication, routes for
  physical objects, odd behavior of,
      (cont.)
    177-181, 197-198, 209-210, 218
      (See also "Paul's lamp")
  sense of presence, 6, 12, 14, 22, 24,
    44-45, 100-104, 106, 111, 113,
    118, 132
  sight, 14 (See more specific headings:
    animal behavior, apparitions,
    lights, etc.)
  smells, 14, 84, 88, 90-98, 163, 189-190
  symbolic events, 14, 43, 64-65,
    136-148
  telepathy, 13-14, 32-46, 101, 111,
    116-117, 137, 161-162, 165, 167
  touch, 14, 19, 44-45, 88, 99-101,
    109-111, 113, 136-137, 161-163,
    178, 190
  visions, 20, 112-113, 193 (See also
    apparitions)
  wind phenomena, 23
after-death communications, seeking
  reconciliation, 102-107, 217, 219
afterlife, denial of, 15, 65
agnosticism, 2
alcoholics and alcoholism, 93, 103-104,
    120, 146, 163, 175, 200-202, 206,
    223
American beliefs regarding the para-
    normal, 61-76, 195
American Psychiatric Association, 64
American religious beliefs and practices,
    59-60, 76
ancestor worship, 5, 49-50
angels, 58, 76, 79, 222
apologies, 102-107, 217, 219
apparitions (See after-death communica-
    tion, routes for)
Arabs, ancient, beliefs and practices,
    54-55
atheism, 2
"atrocity souls," 217 (See also murderers)
authoritarian/angry/abusive upbringing,
    201-202
automatic writing, 166

Balfour, A. J., 28
Balk, David, 10
Barrett, William, 126
battlefield conversion, 93-94
belief in the paranormal, 195-199
bereavement hallucinations (See after-
    death communication)
birds in after-death communication (See
    after-death communication, routes
    for, animal behavior)
blindness, Paul's, 2-4
Boyce, Mary, 68-69
brain development in childhood, 205
Buber, Martin, 22
Buddhist beliefs and practices, 5, 9
butterflies, 152-153

Catholic beliefs and practices, 74
Cayce, Edgar, 199
Celts, ancient, beliefs and practices, 50,
    75-76
Census of Hallucinations, 28-29
childhood influences on sensitivity to the
    paranormal, 196-208 (See also
    stress in childhood)
children, communications from deceased,
    105-114
Chinese beliefs and practices, 49
clairvoyance, 18-19, 21, 63, 144, 194
clocks, 16-19
clouds, 143
Cohn, Shari, 199
Conant, Roberta Dew, 12, 132, 143
crisis apparitions (See death coinci-
    dences) Note: In a crisis appari-
    tion, the perceiver gets an intense
    sense of someone who, around the
    same time, is in a crisis situation
    some distance away. This crisis
    does not necessarily involve a
    death. Death coincidences are one
    form of crisis apparitions.

DCs (See death coincidences)
damnation of the wicked, 56, 59, 73,
    76-77, 217

darkness as an omen of death (*See* after-death communication, routes for)
Days of the Dead, 75
death coincidences (DCs), 16-30, 198
déjà vu, 13
devil, belief in, 76
dissociation, 206
domoviks, 50
Dossey, Larry, 66
Doyle, Sir Arthur Conan, 28
dreams, 73 (*See also* after-death communication, routes for)
dreams, prophetic, role in Old Testament, 72
Duke University parapsychology studies, 17-19
dybbuk, 75

Eastern Orthodox beliefs, 74
Egyptian, ancient beliefs and practices, 52
electromagnetic fields, 115-116
Emmons, Charles, 198
European Human Values Study, 8
evidence, rules of, 68
exorcism, 182-184
extra-sensory perception (ESP), 195-196 (*See also* after-death communication, routes for)

family patterns of sensitivity to psi, 196-199
feeding the dead, 47, 53-54, 58
"fight or flight," 205-206
Flammarion, Camille, 126
flowers and other plants (*See* after-death communication, routes for)
folk wisdom, 68-69
Fundamentalist beliefs, 44, 70-71, 73-75, 77 (*See also* Resurrection)

Gauls, ancient, beliefs and practices, 50
germ theory of disease, 65
Germans, ancient, beliefs and practices, 50
ghosts, 14, 48, 171-178, 180-182, 185-187 (*See also* after-death communication)

God in nature, 213-214
Greeks, ancient, beliefs and practices, 52-53
Greeley, Andrew M., 11, 13
grief, feelings of, as a premonition (*See* after-death communication, routes for)
guardian angels, 58
Guggenheim, Bill and Judy, 12

Hades, 53-54, 57
Halloween, 75-76
Harvard Bereavement Study, 10
Haynes, Renee, 74
hearing (*See* after-death communication, routes for)
heaven, 57, 73-74, 76
hell, 76, 79
help from spirits, 27, 31-46, 118-119, 130-135, 157-171
Hindu beliefs and practices, 4-5, 49
household gods, 50 (*See also* ancestor worship)
Huxley, Thomas Henry, 127

interviews for this book, 13, 61, 195, 211
    Note: A more scholarly report on the author's interview techniques and findings can be found in: Wright, S. H. (1999) "Paranormal contact with the dying: 14 contemporary death coincidences." *Journal of the Society for Psychical Research.* 63 (857) 258-267
intuition, 34
Israelites, ancient, beliefs and practices, 54

James, William, 28
Jehovah's Witnesses, 75
Jenner, Edward, 67-68
Jewish folk beliefs, 22, 75
Jews, ancient, beliefs and practices, 54-55, 57, 72-74
judicial system, 68

Keith (author's son), 2-6
Kikuyu beliefs and practices, 51

LaGrand, Louis E., 12
Last Judgment, 57, 73-75
Lawrence, Tony, 204
levitation, 169
lights (*See* after-death communication, routes for)
Lodge, Sir Oliver, 4, 115-116, 126
log, author's, of paranormal events relating to her personal life, 5, 7-8, 209-210
Luther, Martin, 74

MacGregor, Geddes, 73
Magi, 57
Malinowski, Bronislaw, 48
Mari (Finnish indigenous people), 51
materialism, 15, 76
media images of the paranormal, 14, 61
meditative states, 32, 34, 38, 130-131
mediums and other psychics, 1, 12, 15, 33-34, 54, 63, 66-67, 72, 79-80, 82, 86, 88-90, 97-98, 116, 166, 183-185,194-198, 202-208, 210-219, 223 (*See also* shamans and shamanism)
mental health and after-death communication, 1, 9-13, 61-64 (*See also* reticence about contact experiences)
Mesopotamian beliefs and practices, 52
Mexican beliefs and practices, 75
Montgomery, Ruth, 37
Moody, Raymond, 66, 220
Moslem beliefs and practices, 74
Mount Sinai School of Medicine (New York City), 207
murder victims, 41-42, 164-165
murderers, 217
Murphy, Gardner, 203
mystics and mystical experiences, 47, 64, 79

NORC (*See* National Opinion Research Center)

National Council on Alcoholism and Drug Dependence, 200
National Opinion Research Center, 11
Neanderthals, 47
near-death experiences, 34-35, 47, 63, 66, 220
Newton, Michael, 217

Olson, P. Richard, 10
Orloff, Judith, 64
ouija boards (*See* after-death communication, routes for)
out-of-body experiences, 47, 63
owls, 54-55, 151-152

pagan rituals, 102
parallel psi experiences, 25, 41-46, 105, 107, 114, 116-118, 121, 129, 134, 139, 150-152, 154-155, 163
paranormal, belief in, 195-199
Pasteur, Louis, 65, 67
Paul, the Apostle, 49, 73-74
Paul (author's deceased husband), 2-8
"Paul's lamp," 3-4
Perry, Bruce, 201
physical objects in after-death communication (*See* after-death communication, routes for)
physicists and the paranormal, 4, 28, 35, 115-116, 126
Pike, James A., 133
pituitary gland, 207-208
Playfair, Guy Lyon, 109
polling techniques, limitations of, 13
poltergeists, 133, 178-180
possession, 24, 156-157, 182-187
post-traumatic stress disorder, 206-208
prayer, 21-22, 79, 82
prayer and healing, 66, 71, 163
prayer, answers to, 131
pre-Christian beliefs and practices in Europe, 50
premonitions, 18-19, 144, 168
Protestant beliefs and practices, 74
"psi" defined, 27
psychics (*See* mediums and other psychics)

psychokinesis (PK), 18, 174, 197-198
  (*See also* poltergeists; after-death
  communication, routes for)
puns and wordplay, 2, 6-8
purgatory, 74, 78, 217-222

rainbows, 143
reconciliations via after-death contacts
  (*See* after-death communication
  seeking reconciliation)
Rees, W. Dewi, 9, 73
Reformation, 74
reincarnation, 5, 49, 65, 212
religious beliefs and practices, 2, 13, 21,
  44, 47-60, 195-196, 211-221 (*See
  also* listings under individual faiths
  and national groups)
Remen, Rachel Naomi, 70
remote viewing, 63
resurrection, 73, 75
reticence about contact experiences,
  10-11, 19-20, 61-76
Rhine, Louisa, 18, 30
Richet, Charles, 28
Roberts, Jane, 37
Roman, ancient, beliefs and practices, 53
Rosenblatt, Paul, 47-48

Samhain, 75-76
sanity (*See* mental health)
Santería, 52
Scandinavian folk beliefs and practices, 50
Schwarz, Eitan, 201
scientific method, 34, 67-68
second sight, 19, 198-199 (*See also*
  clairvoyance; premonitions)
sense of presence experiences, nature of,
  131 (*See also* after-death communication, routes for)
Seth Speaks, 37
shamans and shamanism, 9, 15, 50-51,
  64, 69-70, 206
She'ol, 53-54, 57, 221
Shinto faith and practices, 9
Siberian folk beliefs and practices, 50-51
sibling, sensing after-death contact with,
  10

Slavic folk beliefs and practices, 50
smallpox, 67-68
Society for Psychical Research, 28-29,
  115, 126
Spindrift, 66
spirit survival, 5, 49
spirits, unhappy, 25, 217-220
Spiritualism, 97, 126, 168
spirituality, 13, 59-60, 211-215
spirituality, effect on healing, 66
"spontaneous hallucinations of the sane,"
  28
Steiger, Brad, 202-203
Steiner, Rudolf, 199
stress in childhood, 13, 37-38, 93, 146,
  182, 200-208, 223
suicide, 43-45, 77-91
sunsets, 45-46, 143, 153
survival (*See* spirit survival)
symbolic events (*See* after-death
  communication, routes for)

taboos against acknowledging after-death
  communication, 20, 61-76, 194
telepathy 195-196 (*See also* after-death
  communication, routes for)
Tibetan beliefs and practices, 48
touch (*See* after-death communication,
  routes for)
trance (*See* meditative states)
trauma in childhood (*See* stress in
  childhood)
Trobriand Islanders, 48
twins, 109, 197, 199

urine as a cleanser, 68-69

Van Praagh, James, 12
visions (*See* after-death communication,
  routes for)
vitamin C and nitrates, 69

Waldorf school, 105, 199
widows and widowers (*See* after-death
  communication, earlier research
  studies)
Wolff, Robert, 206

Yehuda, Rachel, 207
Yoruba beliefs and practices, 52

Zoroaster and Zoroastrianism, 55-58,
        68-69, 221
Zulu beliefs and practices, 52

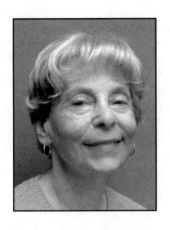

About the Author

Sʏʟᴠɪᴀ Hᴀʀᴛ Wʀɪɢʜᴛ has won numerous academic and literary honors and has been listed in *Who's Who in the East* and *Who's Who of American Women*. A graduate of Cornell University, Professor Wright holds advanced degrees in sociology and information science. Her publications include two books on contemporary American architecture and a monograph on urban education.

Until well into her forties, she had no interest or belief in the paranormal. But after she was widowed in 1983, she began sensing that her husband's spirit was contacting her and learned that others who had been close to him sometimes sensed his presence too. In 1991, Professor Wright retired from the City University of New York, where she headed the library of the School of Architecture and Environmental Studies, and moved to Oregon. Since then she has devoted much of her energy to afterlife research. Articles about her work have appeared in Britain and Italy as well as the United States.

"Over time, my own experiences, plus scores of interviews with people who've had similar ones, have transformed me from a total skeptic to a firm believer in survival of the spirit after death," says Wright. She invites you to check her website at www.spiritscomecalling.com

Aɴᴅʀᴇᴡ Gʀᴇᴇʟᴇʏ, who wrote the foreword, is a distinguished sociologist and bestselling author, as well as a Catholic priest. For over thirty years the director of the Center for the Study of

American Pluralism and a professor at the University of Chicago, his many books include *The Sociology of the Paranormal* and *Religious Change in America.*